PRAISE For
BETTER NOW

NATIONAL BESTSELLER
Longlisted for the BC National Award for Canadian Non-Fiction

"It's a prescription to improve health care across Canada."   —*Healthscape*

"Dr. Martin offers a timely and insightful perspective on Canada's commitment to providing health care as a right to all people. The U.S. health care system has a great deal to learn from Canada and from *Better Now*."
—U.S. Senator Bernie Sanders

"Universal health care is at the very heart of a caring and equitable Canada. Danielle Martin provides us with a practical, accessible and deeply inspiring roadmap for how we can live up to that sacred promise."
—Naomi Klein, author of *This Changes Everything*

"Dr. Danielle Martin has written an outstandingly useful book, for all Canadians, as the nation once again faces the challenges of ensuring effective health care for all. In doing so, Dr. Martin avoids the easy form   of blanket solutions and properly roots health care's future success
choices on delivery, scope, and structure, based on Canadian
—Roy Romanow, former Royal Comm
Future of Health Care in Canada and S
Political Studies, University of Saskatchewan

"A clear-eyed, fearless and detailed manifesto, written with empathy and analytical rigor. For doctors, patients and all Canadians, *Better Now* is an inspiring prescription for the right balance in our shared health care framework."
—Hon. Hugh Segal, Master of Massey College, University of Toronto
and former director of the Institute for Public Policy

BETTER NOW

SIX BIG IDEAS TO IMPROVE
HEALTH CARE FOR ALL CANADIANS

DR. DANIELLE MARTIN

PENGUIN

an imprint of Penguin Canada, a division of Penguin Random House Canada Limited

Penguin Canada
320 Front Street West, Suite 1400, Toronto, Ontario M5V 3B6, Canada

First published in Allen Lane hardcover by Penguin Canada, 2017
Published in this edition, 2018

1 2 3 4 5 6 7 8 9 10

Copyright © 2017 by Danielle Martin

All rights reserved. Without limiting the rights under copyright reserved above, no part of this publication may be reproduced, stored in or introduced into a retrieval system, or transmitted in any form or by any means (electronic, mechanical, photocopying, recording or otherwise), without the prior written permission of both the copyright owner and the above publisher of this book.

Cover and interior design: Jennifer Griffiths
Cover image: Science Photo Library/Getty Images

Printed and bound in the United States of America

Library and Archives Canada Cataloguing in Publication data available upon request

ISBN 978-0-7352-3261-7
eBook ISBN 978-0-7352-3260-0

www.penguinrandomhouse.ca

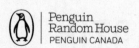

Penguin
Random House
PENGUIN CANADA

CONTENTS

PROLOGUE

In December 1951, after a three-week voyage crossing the Atlantic, my grandfather, Jacques Elie Shilton, reached Pier 21 in Halifax. He was forty-two at the time, and had shepherded ten family members—three generations—through the rigorous and at times perilous process of leaving Egypt for a better life. My mother, who was three, spent the voyage playing with a doll she still remembers.

Gaping at the five-foot-high snowbanks, they boarded the night train for the forty-eight-hour trip to Montreal. My grandparents had left everything behind—their jobs, their savings, their home. They brought several trunks of inappropriate clothing and the few hundred dollars they were allowed to take out of the country. A local immigrant-support organization helped them find an apartment at the outer edge of the city. At least they spoke the language, but the French of North African Jews stuck out as different, just as they did.

My grandfather measured six foot two. He was handsome, with a strong, calm presence and a baritone voice. He spoke seven languages. In Cairo he had worked for a French newspaper, and later for 20th Century Fox. He loved music and he was a talented musician. In the evenings, he played in a dance band to supplement the family income. His two young daughters had no sense of the weight he carried on his shoulders. It seemed to them that he had the strength of ten men.

In the spring of 1953, he went to visit a friend who was being cared for at the Jewish General Hospital in Montreal. But the steep hill on Côte-des-Neiges Road proved too much for him, and as he sat in the waiting room, he suffered a major heart attack. He spent nine weeks in hospital. So began my family's experience of Canadian health care in the pre-medicare days.

After the heart attack, Jacques began having trouble with his breathing. Coughing fits and respiratory distress required frequent visits to the doctor, who had to be paid in cash. Medications were expensive. Sometimes he bought them; at other times, he preferred to save the money. He started having terrible pains in his legs. He experienced increasing difficulty walking, but since every visit to the doctor was expensive, he pushed on.

Time passed, and the pain became unbearable. The blood circulation to his legs was so restricted that his doctor told him his life was on the line. There was no effective treatment for such extensive arterial disease in those days. But then they read about Dr. Michael DeBakey, an international innovator in the emerging field of vascular surgery. DeBakey had pioneered an experimental procedure to open up blood supply in blocked arteries, a technique he hoped could help people with Jacques's problem. He had begun performing it in Houston, Texas. It was worth a shot.

Already crippled by medical debt and his inability to earn a good living, Jacques and my grandmother, Sarah, borrowed money from family members to finance his care, a decision that would taint family relationships for generations. They went to Houston. At my grandfather's request, and in order to save money, the nine-hour surgery was done on both legs at once. During that entire time my grandmother stayed planted on a chair in the waiting room without anyone coming to tell her whether her husband was dead or alive.

Despite the fact that Dr. DeBakey had decided to forgo his fees, Jacques and Sarah couldn't afford to stay in Houston for the recommended six months of convalescence. They returned home nearly immediately.

But the experimental surgery wasn't very successful. The "arteries" that had been inserted served as a pipeline for clots. Jacques was bedridden, and he suffered multiple small heart attacks. He lost fifty pounds and looked like a shadow of the man he had been.

Over the years, the impact on my grandmother was profound. She ate poorly; she had trouble sleeping. The medical bills and the strain of family relationships—ruined now by the borrowed money they couldn't pay back—preyed on her mind. Jacques's efforts to work from his bed, the daily injections of diuretics, the pills, and the constant visits to the doctor wore away at her and her two daughters. Eventually, Sarah's mental health succumbed and she spent six weeks in hospital.

Sarah and Jacques then separated for a time so that they could each try to recover. My mother, who was now in her teens, stayed with Jacques, and her sister went to live with Sarah. The two girls did the best they could to work and contribute to the family income while they embarked on their university studies. And after their mother recovered and was feeling emotionally stronger, Jacques began to court her again. He would bring groceries to her apartment and they would talk about where they might move together in the spring.

But that didn't happen. My mother found him dead at four o'clock in the morning on March 9, 1966, six days after her eighteenth birthday. He was fifty-four years old. He had stayed up more than half the night working on a French-to-English translation to earn a little cash. Sarah, who'd worked from the time they arrived in Canada as an assistant in a fancy Montreal ladies' dress shop, was widowed at age forty-one with a pile of unpaid medical bills on the kitchen table.

My mother's view is that the struggle to deal with financial hardship—along with health problems—destroyed her family. She was studying at McGill at the time, the same university I would attend decades later coming from all the luck and privilege anyone could ask for. She hadn't yet earned her master's degree or launched a successful career. She hadn't yet met my father, a nice boy from a Fine Old Ontario Family who wanted to make the world a better place. She hadn't yet raised a daughter who would make improving health care in Canada her life's passion.

There are more stories of course, but this is a glimpse. It's the story of my family, and also of countless others across Canada who rejoiced when we decided together as a country that it was time to create medicare, a system of hospital and medical care that is free at the point of service for all Canadians.

Health care in Canada isn't perfect. We face very real challenges, challenges I see up close every day. But I grew up believing, as most Canadians do, that the values on which our system is built are sound. That being sick is bad enough without worrying about having to pay for your care. That the families who lived at the top of the hill in Westmount mansions were no more or less deserving of good health care than Jacques and Sarah were.

Our system will need to change to meet the needs of patients over the next fifty years. But that does not require us to institute one system for the rich and another for everyone else. Instead, Canadians can show that we have the courage to address some real and substantial issues without abandoning fairness as if it were a trend that's gone out of fashion.

Most doctors (and nurses, and patients, and citizens) who support medicare are not blind supporters of the status quo. To the extent that our commitment to medicare might make us vulnerable to accepting mediocrity, we need to do better. But we can work for change that addresses our problems and still honours our principles.

As a family doctor working in the system, I believe this now more than ever. Medicare is a work in progress, but it's a work worthy of our greatest efforts. It represents a promise to be the kind of country we can be proud of. This book explains what I think needs to be done to deliver on that promise.

Many books have been written about Canadian health care, and many reports have charted the way forward to improve it. What makes this book any different? It brings together two views that don't always converge: the perspective of the front line—individual patients and health care providers—and the perspective of system thinkers. From that vantage point, I'm proposing six "Big Ideas" for making meaningful improvements to medicare. They focus on cultivating relationship-based primary care, establishing a national drug program, reducing unnecessary and wasteful tests and procedures, reorganizing our existing resources to improve care, ensuring a basic income to promote health, and building the systems we need to actually implement change instead of just talking about it.

As a family doctor, I've had the privilege of working in the Canadian health care system for more than ten years. I have worked in rural northern communities, on First Nation reserves, in small emergency departments and inpatient wards, and downtown in Canada's largest city. My current work is in a general family practice at Toronto's Women's College Hospital, where I teach medical students and residents the art and science of family medicine and see patients of every age and stage. Another part of my practice is taking care of pregnant women and delivering babies. While it sounds trite to say, it's really true that my patients teach me as much about health and health care as I teach them. So throughout these chapters, I'll introduce you to some of the patients who have had a lasting effect on me. I think the lessons of their experience are important to us all. Their names have been changed, and some details of their stories have been altered to protect their privacy. In some cases, these lessons come from colleagues who work in different parts of the health care system and offered case studies of their own memorable patients. All are real people.

————

In addition to my work as a clinician, in my eighth year of practice I started a new job as a vice-president at my hospital. As a medical administrator, I help to manage the hospital budget and to decide what kinds of physicians we need in the hospital. I work on a team that faces tough decisions about how to achieve our hospital's mission within fiscal constraints, how to partner with other organizations in our neighbourhood and beyond, and how to add value for patients in a system under pressure.

When I started this job, Women's College Hospital had committed to redesigning the way we deliver care. Our hospital is different from most: we have no emergency department and no overnight beds. Our maximum length of stay is eighteen hours. We have a large number of general and specialty outpatient clinics; an extensive day-surgery program, including complex surgeries that used to require overnight stays; and a variety of programs for people living with chronic illness. We call ourselves the "hospital designed to keep people out of hospital" because we want to develop new ways of delivering health care to an aging population that wants to live longer, and better, outside an institutional setting. It was that mandate that attracted me to the work.

I had a series of extraordinary mentors who helped prepare me for this job. They encouraged me to take a leadership role at every stage of my career. And with their support and counsel, I did just that. Throughout my medical training, my initial clinical work, and the process of obtaining my master's degree in public policy, I found myself speaking out about the promise of public health care and the need to revitalize our system. In small groups and at conferences, across Canada and the United States, I argued that privatizing some or all of Canadian health care would make us poorer as a society and meaner as a culture. This wasn't solely because of my grandfather's story, although my family's experience remains a sharp reminder of the need for a strong public health care system. It was my work both in health care policy and as a practising doctor that shaped my belief in medicare.

Then one day in early 2014 the phone rang, and everything changed.

THE BASICS

Dr. Martin Goes to Washington

The call came from Bernie Sanders, the long-time Independent congressman and senator from Vermont. He would, of course, later become famous in his spirited run for the Democratic candidacy for president in the 2016 election. His staff knew about the organization I helped found, Canadian Doctors for Medicare—the voice of Canadian doctors who believe in strengthening and improving Canada's publicly funded single-payer system for doctors and hospitals. At that time, I was regularly giving talks at conferences and meetings, writing reports, submitting op-ed pieces to Canadian newspapers, and engaging in public debates with people who favoured privately funded, for-profit solutions to Canada's health care challenges. This seemed like another such presentation—but the source of the invitation sure was different!

As chairman of the U.S. Senate Subcommittee on Primary Health and Aging and a strong advocate for universal health care, Senator Sanders had organized a hearing on what the American health care system could learn from other countries about controlling costs and ensuring universal coverage. Senator Sanders wanted to know: would I come to Washington to talk about what the United States can learn from Canada?

I was honoured and a bit surprised. I accepted his invitation. In the ensuing weeks I went through a standard vetting process: I sent the senator's staff my résumé, and was interviewed by staff members for both Senator Sanders and the senior Republican member of the subcommittee, Senator Richard Burr from North Carolina. I assured them of my academic bona fides and answered their questions about what I was likely to say.

With the help of a terrific policy analyst from Women's College Hospital, Kyla Pollack Behar, who had worked on Capitol Hill, I submitted a written brief in advance of my appearance and drafted my remarks. Then I headed to Washington with Kyla as my guide.

I rehearsed my comments the night before, over and over, alone in my hotel room, timing myself with the stopwatch on my mobile phone. Kyla had warned me that my microphone could be switched off if I went over my five minute time allotment. The following morning I was standing outside the Senate building, at the end of a very long lineup, forty minutes before the hearing was scheduled to begin.

"These guys need a wait-times strategy," I texted Kyla, who was waiting inside for me. I'd been looking on as the people in line were slowly screened, one by one. There was a huge bottleneck at the one screening machine, where bored-looking security staff stood back and watched one person do most of the work. I worried about arriving late for the hearing. Meanwhile, I could see through the lobby to the other side of the building, where a second entrance—also staffed by security guards—stood empty.

I made it into the hearing with seconds to spare, and sat down at a long table alongside other presenters who'd been invited to speak about their nations' health care systems. We each had five minutes to discuss what the United States could learn from Denmark, Taiwan, France, and Canada, and then there would be a question-and-answer period.

I had two simple goals heading into that Senate session.

First, I wanted to stand up for the values that underpin the Canadian health care system, without being an apologist for it.

Of course our system has problems, and I wasn't there to defend the indefensible. My role was to explain what we're doing in Canada to address our problems, and why we want to do that without giving up on the principle of fairness that defines our publicly funded system. I needed to walk that line between sticking up for Canadian medicare and defending the status quo.

Second, I wanted to keep my cool. I understood that this was political theatre. The senators weren't really talking *to* each other but *over* each other in a conversation that was taking place as much for an audience outside the room as inside it. I had a small cameo in a much larger performance. I needed to stay composed and play the role assigned to me, knowing that nothing I could say in a brief presentation would change anyone's mind in the American health care debate.

My remarks ended just shy of my allotted five minutes. There were a few heated moments in the Q&A, but I felt good about how I handled them. Soon the two hours were over and Kyla and I were headed back to the airport.

On the flight home, I told Kyla that I thought the session had gone really well in terms of my two goals. "It's too bad no one back home will ever know about it," I said. "Do you think if I wrote one, *Maclean's* would publish an article about what it's like to be a Canadian doctor who gets grilled about our health care system by U.S. senators?" She shrugged in a way that gently suggested most people wouldn't be very interested, and I had to agree.

The following evening, as I was heading home from the hospital clinic, my phone started to buzz. Then it buzzed again, and again, with text messages and voicemail from people who'd seen clips of the hearing. It didn't stop buzzing for about three weeks. Everyone I knew was telling me that they were watching or listening to those clips. I was on CTV. MSNBC. CBC. Radio. TV. Trending on Twitter. On Facebook. On Yahoo News. "You're breaking the internet!" a friend texted. The next day my face was on the front page of the *Toronto Star* (and so was Kyla's, sitting right behind me).

The entire hearing had been filmed, as are all hearings of the U.S. Senate. Within hours of my departure from Washington, Senator

Sanders's staff had posted a clip on YouTube of a particularly biting exchange between Republican Senator Richard Burr and me. The *Los Angeles Times* picked it up under the headline "Watch an Expert Teach a Smug U.S. Senator About Canadian Health Care"—and the next thing I knew, the clip was everywhere.

The video that landed me on the front pages of Canadian and international news media culminated in the following exchange:

SENATOR BURR: Dr. Martin . . . why are doctors exiting the public system in Canada?

DR. MARTIN: Thank you for your question, Senator . . . in fact we see a net influx of physicians from the United States into the Canadian system over the last number of years. What I did say was that the solution to the wait-time challenge that we have in Canada . . . does not lie in moving away from our single-payer system towards a multi-payer system . . . Australia used to have a single-tier system, and in the 1990s moved to a multiple-payer system where private insurance was permitted. A very well-known study . . . [found that] in those areas of Australia where private insurance was being taken up and utilized, waits in the public system became longer.

SENATOR BURR: What do you say to an elected official who goes to Florida and not the Canadian system to have a heart valve replaced?

DR. MARTIN: . . . In fact the people who are the pioneers of that particular surgery which Premier Williams had . . . are in Toronto at the Peter Munk Cardiac Centre, just down the street from where I work. So what I say is that sometimes people have a perception— and I believe that actually this is fuelled in part by media discourse—that going to where you pay more for something, that that necessarily makes it better. But it's not actually borne out by the evidence on outcomes for that cardiac surgery or any other.

. . .

SENATOR BURR: Dr. Martin, in your testimony you state that the focus should be on reducing waiting times in a way that is equitable for all. What length of time do you consider to be equitable when waiting for care?

DR. MARTIN: Well, in fact the Wait Time Alliance in Canada, sir, has established benchmarks across a variety of different diagnoses for what's a reasonable period to wait. . . . You know, I waited more than thirty minutes at the security line to get into this building today, and when I arrived in the lobby I noticed across the hall that there was a second entry point with no lineup whatsoever. Sometimes it's not actually about the amount of resources that you have but rather about how you organize people in order to use your queues most effectively. And that's what we're working to do because we believe that when you try to address wait times you should do it in a way that benefits everyone, not just people who can afford to pay.

SENATOR BURR: On average, how many Canadian patients on a waiting list die each year? Do you know?

DR. MARTIN: I don't, sir, but I know that there are forty-five thousand in America who die waiting because they don't have insurance at all.

The ensuing weeks were a blur. I received emails and letters from all over the world. I was interviewed by media wanting the back story. I was called a "national hero" by people who liked my message and "Joan of Arc" by people who didn't. I was stopped in the street and the grocery store. The speaking invitations started rolling in. The chief of surgery at my hospital said to me, "You should write a book."

Of course it was fun to experience those few minutes of fame, but it was also informative. I had touched a nerve.

From that groundswell of support and media attention, I came to the following conclusion. Many, many Canadians still care deeply about—in fact are wildly proud of—our publicly funded health care system, what we call medicare. (The same name is used to describe the American public insurance system that covers people over age sixty-five.) In poll after poll, medicare is cited as our most defining social program. Its importance to our national psyche is indisputable: in a 2012 Leger Marketing poll, 94 percent of those surveyed said it was an important source of both personal and collective pride.

I fully grasped the intensity of that enthusiasm for public health care only when—for a brief moment—it was directed at me. It is not an exaggeration to say that for many people across this country, medicare *is* what it means to be Canadian. It strengthens our economy, improves our social stability, and exemplifies our values.

That's the dual promise of medicare. To deliver accessible, high-quality services in an equitable way. And to give us something to be proud of.

This dual promise means that to improve medicare, we need to think not only about better delivery of services—a promise that is hard enough to keep—but also about making it a social program worthy of its iconic status. Medicare should still inspire us.

The "iconic" nature of Canadian health care is not news. Indeed, it's often discussed, sometimes in a derisive way, in books and articles about health care system reform. Some of this commentary claims that our commitment to the principles of medicare prevents us from improving the system—because we're blinded to its imperfections and because we're afraid that any change at all will drive us into American-style, for-profit health care. We can't, the argument goes, see our way to solutions, because doing so would require us to change an iconic program, the political cost of which would be too great. Through this lens, Canadian pride in our health care system appears stubbornly childish, a barrier to what some call the "adult discussion" we need to have about the future of health care.

I disagree. The fact that Canadians are deeply committed to medicare isn't an impediment to change. Our commitment is—or should be—the *foundation* for change. This was what former premier Roy Romanow meant when he called his report on the future of health care "Building on Values." Having a commitment to the value of equity isn't childish. The notion that a social program like publicly funded, universal health insurance has become a symbol of our nation is something we can be proud of—as long as it doesn't cause us to rest on our laurels. We won't turn our backs on the basic structure of the program or sacrifice our principles. We don't have to. Instead, we need to address the challenges in health care in ways that build on what's good about what we already have in place.

I haven't done every job in the health care system. I'm not a surgeon or a subspecialist. I've never worked outside Ontario. But I do think that my current roles as a practising doctor, a hospital administrator, and an advocate have helped me see at least some of what works and what doesn't work in our health care system.

Peter Selby, a Toronto family doctor with expertise in public health and mental health care, once suggested to me that to see health care clearly, we need "bifocal vision." One lens must focus on what has to be done right up close, at the level of the individual patient sitting in a doctor's office needing help. The other lens must focus at a distance, giving us a long-range, overall perspective on the system. Through that lens, the population—not the individual—is the unit of analysis. I hope that this book will offer both lenses: a bifocal vision for the future of Canada's most cherished social program.

Getting Our Facts Straight

Health care systems are structurally fairly simple. As my grandfather, Jacques, knew all too well, someone has to pay for the care. That's called health care financing. And someone has to give the care to patients. That's called delivery. If you understand who's paying for the service and who's delivering it, you can begin to understand the health care model being discussed.

Health care can be financed publicly or privately, or through a combination of both public and private money. Public financing in Canada comes primarily through tax dollars: we all put money into the pot through our taxes, and then our federal and provincial governments use that money to pay for our care. The money is distributed through our public plans, one in each province and territory and others at the federal level. The plans then pay for the care we receive. Examples of publicly financed health care include any service for which you use your health card: a visit to your family doctor, an admission to the hospital, a chest X-ray. About 70 percent of Canadian health care is paid for from the public purse. On the financing side, for most hospital and physician care, we have a *single payer*—the public insurance plan—in each province.

This public insurance plan, of course, is what was missing in my grandfather's day, and what is still missing today in countries all over the world. When no publicly financed system exists, the only option is private financing. In Jacques's case, this meant begging family members to help pay for his care.

In today's Canada, privately financed care—care paid for through means other than your tax dollars—accounts for 30 percent of health spending. This includes services that are covered through private supplemental insurance (such as employee benefit plans) as well as those that you have to dig into your wallet to pay for. Most dental care and prescription drugs and much physiotherapy and psychotherapy are examples of privately financed care.

In my day-to-day work, it matters a great deal what is publicly financed and what is privately financed. This is because services that are publicly financed are accessible for all my patients (although if a patient has to wait a long time, then these services aren't as accessible as they should be). If a patient needs a surgeon to remove her gallbladder, I don't have to ask whether she can afford to pay for it, or whether she has insurance, and whether that insurance covers gallbladders. I just refer her to any general surgeon, because I know that medically necessary surgery is covered for everyone with a health card.

On the other hand, when I worked in hospitals in rural northern Ontario, I often saw people come into the emergency department with dental abscesses. One man's face and neck were so swollen from infection that I was afraid it would obstruct his airway and prevent him from breathing. He'd had an infected tooth for months. But because he didn't have dental coverage, and couldn't afford to pay, he hadn't gone to the dentist.

In Canada, every province has established a single-payer insurance scheme for "medically necessary medical care services," which has essentially come to mean most things that take place in a hospital or are done by a doctor. These insurance plans cover all eligible residents, and they function on a not-for-profit basis. (A small but not insignificant number of people are not eligible, usually due to their immigration status.) Any province that violates the principles of the Canada Health

Act—which requires the single-payer scheme for those services—is at risk of having the federal government claw back dollars from its share of the funding allocation.

There are two reasons why Canada has chosen the single-payer model of health insurance.

The first is equity, or fairness. With only one payer, the queue for treatment is ordered on the basis of need, not ability to pay. If Jacques were alive today and unable to walk, he would not have to worry about paying for his care. He would be offered the available treatments according to his level of need—though perhaps not the kind of extremely experimental treatment he ultimately underwent when his problem had progressed to the end stage.

Perfect equity does not exist in the Canadian health care system, nor in any other. But a system that covers everyone and does not permit systematized preferential access for the wealthy or better insured is as close as any system can come. And despite what critics say, such a system does not necessarily, and should not, lead to long wait times.

The second reason we have a single-payer system for doctors and hospitals in Canada—a reason that doesn't get enough attention, in my view—is that these systems are much less administratively expensive than the alternatives.

As a doctor, I send one bill to one insurance company once a month—the Ontario Health Insurance Plan—and I get paid every month, on time. Better yet, my patients don't have to go to an accounts office to pay their bills and then seek reimbursement from an insurance company. Compare this to the complexity of administration in multi-payer systems: insurance companies must develop benefit packages, explain them to potential users, market them against the competition, evaluate applications for insurance, assess and pay claims, and, in the case of investor-owned companies, turn a profit each year for their shareholders. Our medicare plans bear almost none of these costs. As the single payer, OHIP has prices that are centrally negotiated. The plan requires no marketing, and it has no profit incentive.

The complexity and overhead involved in multi-payer financing systems explains why American private insurance companies spend an estimated 18 percent of the premiums they bring in on billing and insurance-related administration. By contrast, Canada's elegantly simple single-payer system spends less than 2 percent on insurance overhead for the public plans found in each province and territory.

Having multiple payers, including private insurers, will always raise administrative costs. We see examples of this all around the world, including right here in Canada. Administrative costs are a lot higher for things covered through private insurance, such as prescription drugs, than for health services covered by provincial single payers, such as doctors' services and hospital care.

Who pays for the service—the financing—matters so much. It's separate from who delivers the service—which also matters, but in a different way.

———

Health care is publicly *delivered* when the government directly supplies services to patients. In that situation, those who are delivering the care, such as doctors and nurses, are government employees. One example of this in Canada is public health departments. The people who manage outbreaks of infectious disease and run our immunization programs are usually public employees. → doctors are paid privately

But aside from public health departments, we have almost no public delivery in Canada. In fact, we have a highly private health care delivery system. That hasn't changed much since the pre-medicare days. When my grandfather went to see a doctor in an office down the street from his Montreal apartment, that doctor was an independent entrepreneur. He charged Jacques directly, whereas today he would have charged the government of Quebec for his services. Yet the doctor's status as an independent—or "private"—practitioner would today differ little from what it was in the 1950s.

Most of our publicly financed health care services—those paid for with tax dollars—are still privately delivered. This is a really important point, often misunderstood. As a doctor, I'm paid with public dollars, but I'm not an employee of the government. When I see a patient, the single payer (in my case, OHIP) deposits the money for my fee into my account, but I'm still self-employed.

The minister of health is not my boss. Because I'm paid as an independent contractor for my services, the minister can't mandate that I work evening hours, for example, or correspond with my patients by email. He or she can't fire me, because like nearly all Canadian physicians, I'm not a government employee. If they want me to practise medicine differently, policy makers in the Ministry of Health could entice me to do so by paying a premium for any patient seen after five p.m., or conversely, by cutting the rates for daytime consultations. This is very different from other health care systems—such as the English and the Scottish National Health Service—where hospital-based physicians like me are under much more direct control from the state, primarily because they're actually public employees.

So provincial governments don't deliver health care directly, but they do try to use their dollar power to shape the way doctors and hospitals deliver care.

The distinctions don't end there. Not all privately delivered health care is the same.

Imagine that you need to pick up a few items for your home—toothpaste and dish soap, maybe. You have options. Perhaps you're a member of a co-op and like to do your shopping there. Or you might walk to your local corner store, owned by a family that lives in your neighbourhood. You could drive to a large, independently owned store in your community. Finally, you could choose a big-box store, a multinational chain that looks the same in Calgary as it does in Texas.

The same kinds of distinctions exist in health care delivery. Is a "private" doctor's office, with a few physicians practising together and sharing overhead costs, the same thing as a multinational chain that owns hundreds of clinics and delivers annual dividends to its shareholders? Of course not. Private delivery exists on a spectrum.

At one end of the spectrum is private, not-for-profit delivery, as in many Canadian hospitals. As a hospital administrator myself, I can vouch for the fact that the boards and administrators who run Ontario hospitals are acutely aware of what the government wants from us, but our hospitals are not owned or operated directly by that government, and we are not employees of the Ministry of Health. Hospital care is, therefore, usually publicly financed, in a model of *private, not-for-profit* delivery.

At the other end of the spectrum are for-profit corporations that deliver health care. They might be single organizations, domestically owned chains, or even multinational corporations. In Canada we see them most often in the provision of community laboratory services, nursing homes, and home care, though in recent years more for-profit primary care and even for-profit surgical centres have been cropping up. These organizations may be providing publicly financed care—paid for with tax dollars—but they're private, for-profit, investor-owned, shareholder-driven companies. They are the big-box equivalents—in fact, sometimes they're even located right inside big-box stores.

Many models of health care delivery exist somewhere between those two ends of the spectrum, such as when doctors work in "private practice." This is for-profit delivery, of course: physicians want to earn an excess of revenue (their clinical billings) over expenses (such as paying a secretary, starting a filing system, renting an office) so that they can take the rest home in wages. But because this isn't a large, investor-owned business, it's best described as the "for-profit small business" model. This has traditionally been the dominant model in Canada, especially in family medicine and for specialists outside hospitals.

When people talk about Canada having a "government monopoly" over health care services, they misunderstand our system. In fact, nearly all our health care is privately delivered, and, as I mentioned earlier, fully 30 percent of our health care services are privately financed. Those who use words like "monopoly" are really objecting to the fact that each province and territory has only one payer for doctors and hospitals and Canadians can't buy their way to the front of the line. This is exactly as it should be to ensure equitable access. When some can pay and some can't, as occurs in a "two-tier" design, equity is compromised, or abandoned.

"Two-tier" health care is a confusing term that can have different meanings. People sometimes say that we already have a two-tier system because now and again professional baseball players get faster access to MRI scans than bakers do.

It's true, of course, that we don't have perfect equity in Canada. For example, we know that women have more difficulty accessing some services than men. People in rural communities, those living in poverty, Indigenous people, and other marginalized groups don't experience the same access to health care that educated urban people do. The reasons for this are complex, but they're not related to cost as a barrier to access at the point of care. It may be that even today under medicare, my grandfather, who was a Jewish, brown-skinned, first-generation francophone immigrant, would have experienced trouble getting the same care that a bank CEO receives. But under a single-payer, universal model like the one we have now, his chances would have been a lot better.

A true two-tiered system is one in which people pay privately to gain access to health care services more quickly or in an environment they perceive to be "better." They might pay directly, out of their pockets, for that care, or they might purchase private insurance coverage. "Two tier" refers to parallel public and private financing systems whereby people can purchase with private money the same services they could get in the publicly financed system. Such systems exist in many other countries, including England and Australia. We don't have that in Canada.

And yet some people occasionally leverage social networks to get faster or "better" care. For no additional cost, knowing someone who works inside the health care system may help with navigating care, and not everyone has access to this type of social capital. I sometimes see this in my practice, when patients call or email me to say that they've arranged an appointment for themselves next week with a specialist who's the friend of a friend (and who has a six-month waiting list). Would I mind faxing over a referral?

I do mind, of course, because it feels so unfair when that person's problem isn't urgent, but yes, I've done it anyway, when I didn't know how else to preserve my relationship with my patient. Most of us know of someone who was able to get quick access to something they didn't need urgently, because their aunt is a secretary in the hospital or they have a friend who's a surgeon. That doesn't mean we have a two-tier health care system, although it does illustrate the reality that no system is beyond gaming. We design systems to work for most of us, most of the time, and that don't discriminate against people with big needs and few resources. It might be possible to plug all the holes that allow inappropriate preferential access, but it would require a huge input of energy. Just ask the Canada Revenue Agency what it's like to stay ahead of clever people who play the annual tax avoidance game.

There is no systematic way for patients in Canada to purchase faster or better care than someone else who has greater need. As a physician, I can't legally take money or basketball tickets from patients to help them jump the queue. So where there are problems, rather than just exiting the system, we're all going to have to work together to fix them—not just for a few, but for everybody. This requires us to understand the structures within which change will take place.

———

Canada's federal system of government has shaped the development of medicare. Our Constitution establishes a division of powers between the federal and provincial/territorial governments. This division determines which level of government is responsible for the different areas of policy that affect health.

The delivery of health care services is constitutionally under provincial jurisdiction. Our provinces and territories have primary responsibility for managing most of our health care systems. The federal government doesn't deliver health care services to most Canadians, but it does provide money to support health care in every province and territory.

Despite that constitutional division of powers, the federal government is essential to protecting and improving medicare. As well as setting standards for what the provinces must do in return for federal dollars, the federal government can use its spending power to shape the provincial insurance plans.

The big tool that the federal government has used to shape how the provinces deliver care is the Canada Health Act, which was unanimously passed into law in 1984. In order to receive federal funding for health care, provinces have to adhere to principles of the CHA, including not allowing doctors or hospitals to charge patients extra for services covered by medicare.

In addition to this, agreements called Health Accords have at times been negotiated between the premiers and the prime minister to determine joint priorities for health care improvement. These then become areas where additional (or even existing) federal dollars are directed. This is sometimes referred to as federal funding with "strings attached"—meaning that, rather than the federal government just issuing a cheque to the provinces, national investments are directed toward shared priorities.

Such accords have addressed issues like immunizations for children and wait times for joint replacements and cataract surgery. Today or in the future, priority areas that could be addressed under a Health Accord might include a national approach to improving home and community care, national pharmacare, or a national plan to improve access to mental health care for both children and adults. Of course, this depends on the federal government's willingness to use the tax revenue it collects to drive change in any of these areas.

When it comes to Indigenous health care in Canada, the system is complicated. For on-reserve First Nations and Inuit communities, the federal government has traditionally financed *and* delivered health services. At the same time, First Nation peoples and Inuit are covered under provincial and territorial medicare plans. This can create divided systems of care in which access to, and the continuity of, care can be problematic—which is one reason, among many important others, why Indigenous peoples in Canada continue to have much worse health outcomes than the general population. There are higher rates of chronic and contagious diseases in these communities and, on the whole, a shorter life expectancy—problems of grave concern to us all.

Arrangements between the federal government, the provinces, and those delivering health care on the ground are complex, and their relationship to health outcomes is even more complex. But if you understand who pays for the service and who delivers it, you can begin to make sense of the issues. The next time someone starts telling you that they're for or against "private health care," your first question should be "Are you talking about financing or delivery?"

———

I recognize that not everyone is as interested in the difference between financing and delivery as I am. The truth is that, when I graduated from medical school in 2003, I didn't know much about these things. I knew I had to understand the larger picture—not only the causes of disease under the microscope but also how a health system is planned, managed, and paid for—but I hadn't had training in those system-level issues. I find that not much has changed: many residents graduating and launching their practices today don't have a very clear sense of what makes medicare work.

For physicians, the rules that govern medicare are important because they're rules that affect how we practise medicine. All health care systems place limits on the behaviour of doctors, and ours is no exception. In Canada, there are two major restrictions on physicians.

First, doctors are not allowed to "extra bill" patients, the practice of charging more than what the provincial plan pays doctors for necessary services. As a physician, I can't ask my patients to pay me more than what

OHIP would pay for a consultation. In other words, I don't set the price for my services. It's set in negotiations between the government and the medical association. (Of course, for services *not* covered by medicare, such as cosmetic services, doctors can charge whatever the market will bear.)

Second, doctors are prevented from conducting a dual practice. Canadian physicians and surgeons cannot see patients in the publicly funded system on Monday and then see patients who pay out of pocket for insured services on Tuesday. We're either working in the public system or we're not. This makes it more burdensome for doctors to exit the public system, because to do so we have to unenroll entirely from medicare, thus eliminating what would otherwise be a core, and reliable, income source.

These controls on the billing practices of doctors are partly (actually, in large measure) what makes medicare tick. By reducing the financial incentives for physicians to exit the public system—usually without actually making it illegal to do so—governments have created a structure where it is unappealing to most doctors to work outside the public health care system.

You might think these controls would result in low incomes for Canadian physicians, especially since doctors in countries with two-tier systems often supplement their incomes substantially by seeing "private patients." Instead, Canadian physicians are among the best-paid doctors in the world. A 2015 report from the Organisation for Economic Co-operation and Development (OECD) found that Canadian general practitioners or family doctors bring in nearly three times the average Canadian income. Specialists bring in over four and a half times that average income. While such rankings often don't take administrative overhead costs (which can be significant) into account, the fact remains that Canadian doctors are well paid for the work they do. This is part of what helps protect us against a "brain drain" of doctors south of the border, a problem we haven't had for many years.

———

The basic structure of our system is not always well understood by those who offer prescriptions for health care reform in Canada. Yet that context is crucial. By understanding the roles of our governments, the difference between financing and delivery, the limits on physicians, and the rationale for our single-payer design, we can begin to answer the critical question of how to make health care in Canada better.

Taking the Pulse of the System

This book is about making medicare better. But "better" in health care is a tricky word. Better in what way? Longer lives for Canadians? A better experience travelling through the system when we get sick? More affordable care? Health care systems don't have just one goal. They aim to deliver health *and* a good experience to patients—at a cost we can all afford.

The notion that health care systems have to achieve all these things at once was a light-bulb moment for many when it was first articulated clearly. The term *Triple Aim* was coined in 2008 by Dr. Don Berwick and his colleagues at the Institute for Healthcare Improvement in the United States. They said that if we want to improve quality in health care, we need to do three things simultaneously: first, improve the health of the population; second, improve the patient experience of care; and third, lower (or hold constant) the per capita cost of care so that the health care system can be sustainable.

Whenever we implement a new way of delivering care, we should be measuring our success across all three aspects of the Triple Aim. Instead of seeking innovations that do just one of these things—like cool health apps that people enjoy but don't actually improve health, or very expensive drugs that extend life minimally but reduce quality of life—we should aim for all three simultaneously.

Sound impossible? It isn't. But it does require focus.

So, how are we doing in our quest to achieve the Triple Aim in Canadian medicare?

The first goal in the Triple Aim is to improve the health of the population. And at the population level, our health is generally quite good—with the noted exceptions of Indigenous peoples and some other marginalized groups. The proportion of Canadians who say they are in good or excellent health is high, which is great news. Our average life expectancy is just over eighty-one years, one year ahead of the average among developed countries, and our infant mortality rates inch just above average.

But those statistics aren't the best measure of a health care system. Life expectancy is more related to social factors like poverty and education than it is to the performance of our doctors and hospitals. The test of how a system performs is how well we're doing on outcomes for diseases that we know are treatable. For example, deaths from bacterial infections, diabetes, treatable cancers, cardiovascular disease, or even complications from surgical procedures are measures that better tell the story of a health system's performance. By this measure, Canada comes in sixth place among nineteen high-income peer countries.

Taken disease by disease, we can see how we do in even more detail. When compared to thirty-four OECD countries, we ranked second last (very well) in deaths from stroke, nineteenth in deaths from heart disease, and thirteenth in deaths due to cancer. Overall, I would give our health care system a B for outcomes.

If your child comes home from school with a B grade, the first thing you'll probably want to check is whether he's improving compared to the last report card. A student who got a C last semester and earned a B this time deserves praise. An A-student who got a B needs a sit-down.

But what if you don't know how he did last semester? What you may not realize is that the people delivering health care in Canada often have no idea about the quality of care they're providing, or whether we're doing any better this year than last year.

We collect lots of data in Canadian health care, but we do a very poor job of putting information about how we're doing into the hands of providers and patients. Few surgeons know their complication rates or how those rates compare to those of their colleagues; few family doctors know how long their patients are waiting to get an appointment; and almost no one is getting paid based on the quality of care they're providing. If there's something to the old adage that you can't manage what you don't measure, we clearly aren't doing enough to support improvement of health care quality in Canada. Which makes it really hard to know what grade we deserve and whether we're on the right track for improvement.

Part of the reason for this gap is that our information technology systems aren't up to snuff. Over the last ten years we've done much better in moving away from paper, but we continue to have problems with the integration of our digital systems. Just because the hospital and the family doctor's office both use computers doesn't mean that those computers talk to each other. Our information systems aren't yet able to pull this week's data so that providers can do better for patients next week, nor are patients able to routinely gain access to their own health data. In the absence of that kind of measurement and reporting, it's hard to improve the outcomes of the care we deliver.

———

Of course, the big political controversy in Canada over whether medicare delivers the goods isn't really about the outcomes once people get into the system. It's about access. Timely access is especially important to people's experience of care—the second part of the Triple Aim— though it can also influence both the health of the population and the cost of care if it's seriously and consistently compromised.

Access to a wait list isn't access to care. Many patients in my practice wait months for elective surgery or to see a specialist for a non-urgent problem. Our system does a terrific job of delivering care when people are seriously ill, and most of us are otherwise prepared to accept some amount of waiting. But we have a lot of work to do to reduce wait times in Canada for non-urgent but still necessary medical care.

Think back to the last time you were sick and needed to see your doctor. When you called for an appointment, could you be seen within forty-eight hours? Unfortunately, fewer than half of Canadians report that they could. Nearly one in five Canadians who needs elective (not urgent) surgery will wait longer than four months for it; that number is unacceptably high compared to other developed countries. The methods used to compare health care in different countries are always criticized, and there's often a good basis for those criticisms. But for anyone who works in the Canadian health care system or has needed care of a non-urgent nature, the general findings ring true.

This is a problem that can be fixed. We can learn to do better, and we have. In some areas we've seen improvements on wait times. According to the annual Wait Time Alliance report cards, between 2012 and 2013, Canada went from an A to an A+ on waits for radiation oncology, which means that nearly everyone is treated within the four-week benchmark time frame. From 2013 to 2014, the B and C on hip and knee replacements improved to an A and B, respectively.

The good thing about our wait-times problem is that it isn't a problem when needs are critical. In my experience as a Canadian family doctor, in both rural communities and big cities, if I pick up the phone to get something for a patient who really needs it, the system nearly always moves. If it's an emergency or highly urgent, my patient is not going to wait. Sometimes she may need me to advocate and navigate the system for her, which is what family physicians are supposed to do. But in those critical moments, Canadians get the care they need, and the care they get is usually very good.

But what if my patient is a lawyer who experiences bothersome (but not life-threatening) headaches, isn't responding to the usual treatments, and misses a day a week of work while waiting weeks or months for his neurology appointment? Or a grandmother who forfeits a whole golf season waiting for her hip surgery? Or a child showing early signs of a developmental disability who loses a semester waiting for an assessment? These people are not in "life or limb" danger, but the effects of waiting are real, and the waits need to be addressed.

The problem with the wait-times debate in Canada is this: some people want to introduce private financing into our physician and hospital systems in order to either support their free-market ideology or garner personal profit. They've seized on wait times as a justification, arguing that it's single-payer, publicly funded medicare that engenders long wait lists. But those two things—wait times and private financing—have nothing to do with each other.

Some countries with single-tier systems have long waits, and some have short waits. Some countries with two-tier systems have long waits, and some have short waits. Our wait time problem isn't caused by the fact that we pay for our health care collectively instead of individually. It's mainly caused by poor organization of the resources we have.

Long waits affect real people, and they need to be addressed—not by massively increasing our health spending but by better organizing our resources. If we could do that, we would greatly improve Canadians' experience of the health care system.

———

Reducing costs, or holding them constant, is the third aspect of the Triple Aim. We already spend a lot of money on health care in Canada, as do all developed nations. In 2013 (the latest year for which data are available at the time of writing), we spent nearly 11 percent of our GDP on health care services, putting us in the top quarter of OECD countries in terms of health care spending per person. The same percentage is expected to have been spent in 2015.

Some people say that this means we have an expensive health care system. That's true if they're talking about *total* expenditures, which include public spending on things like doctors and hospitals as well as private spending on things like dentists and prescription drugs. But among developed countries, the proportion of our health spending that's *public* is near the bottom. For every dollar we spend on health care in Canada, seventy cents comes from government. Compare this to the U.K., where eighty-three cents of the average health care dollar is publicly financed. In Norway, it's eighty-five cents. In France, it's seventy-nine cents. It's only because we so often compare ourselves to the United States, which has the highest private spending (48 percent) and the lowest public spending (52 percent) on health care in the developed world, that we tend to think of our public spending on health care as being high. By international standards, it is not.

Canadians spend a lot of money buying private insurance and paying out of pocket for services not covered by medicare. We have very low levels of public funding for essential services like prescription medications (about 40 percent) and dental services (about 5 percent), not to mention home care, physiotherapy, and long-term care. Since 1998, our average out-of-pocket health care expenses have been rising much faster than inflation. As a result, increasing numbers of Canadian families are spending substantial amounts of their incomes on services like dental care and prescription medicines. For too many, that means choosing between medical necessities and other necessities, like rent or food. A sustainable system is one that is affordable not just for governments, but also for citizens.

Indeed, if you follow the news on Canadian health care, you know that the word "sustainability" now makes its way into virtually every conversation, often in the context of doomsday predictions. Usually, the argument sounds something like this: "Twenty years ago health care took up only 26 percent of our provincial budget. Today it takes up 43 percent. If we continue along these lines, soon we won't have any money available for schools, roads, or anything else—our entire government will just be one big Ministry of Health." This has been called the Pac-Man argument—I always picture a big health care Pac-Man eating up all the other social services in the lanes it travels through.

There are many things wrong with the Pac-Man analysis. The first is what's been called the "straight lines of death" fallacy—the belief that since health care costs have grown in the past, they'll continue to grow at the same rate in the future. Yet this is untrue: the early 2000s saw a long-term upward trend in health care expenditures, but just as people started to panic, governments reined in spending growth following the 2008–2009 recession. Our total spending on health care is now *falling* as a proportion of GDP—hardly a "straight line of death."

The second thing wrong with the Pac-Man analysis is its tricky math. While health care costs were rising in the past few decades, provincial budgets were shrinking. The best way to illustrate this point is through a story that Dr. Michael Rachlis, a public health specialist in Toronto, likes to tell.

> Imagine there's a family of four living together in a small house— two adults and their two kids. Every evening they have dinner together. One September the older child, now eighteen years old, goes off to university. For several weeks the remaining three family members continue their family meal each evening. But one evening the parents sit down with the younger child and say, "Son, we're very sorry but we can't afford to keep you around anymore. Last year you were eating only 25 percent of the food in this house. Now you're eating 33 percent of it!"

This is what has happened in health care. Of course the younger son isn't eating any more than he ate before his brother left. Rather, the denominator has gone from four people to three. As governments across the country cut taxes over the last two decades, the size of the communal pie—the total budget for public services—began to shrink. This made the fraction—health care spending as a portion of the total budget—appear to grow impressively.

No one likes to cut health care, so it's been (mostly) shielded from cuts. Instead, cuts were made to social assistance, to colleges and universities, or to programs for new immigrants. This isn't the fault of the health care system. We should value and protect the other important programs we choose to fund with our tax dollars. But we shouldn't have to choose between health care and roads unless we're prioritizing tax cuts over both health care and roads. In this scenario, the Pac-Man devouring things isn't health care—it's tax cuts. And these days, as citizens have pushed for better public services, governments are having to rethink tax cuts.

The third problem with the Pac-Man analysis (and another frequent cause of front-page hysteria about health system sustainability) is the myth that our aging population will drive health care costs through the roof. Let me emphasize: *our aging population will not bankrupt the health care system*. Well, at least not by simply aging. The proportion of Canadians over the age of sixty-five is increasing, but here's the thing about aging: it happens only one year at a time.

It's true that we use more health care services as we age, but as Canadian economist Bob Evans has so eloquently put it, we aren't facing a grey tsunami but rather a very slowly moving grey glacier. If Canadian seniors continue to use health care at the same rates they currently do—which includes higher use as they age and especially in the final weeks of life—we can expect to see health care costs grow by about 1 percent per year (depending on the province) as seniors move through the system. Even modest economic growth should be able to absorb that kind of increase.

The real challenge of an aging population isn't the increasing number of aging baby boomers, but the increasing number of tests and treatments we administer to them *without improving their health*.

If people in the future use about the same amount of health care as their equivalents do today, we need not fear the aging population. But if usage rates don't remain constant, costs will increase faster than we think, regardless of how old people are. The biggest increase in health care costs over the last decade has come not from aging but from increased use of hospitals, drugs, and doctors.

Every Canadian adult, *of every age group*, is using more health care than his or her equivalent did twenty years ago. This includes heavier and more intense treatment even for healthy people over the age of sixty-five, not just those with chronic illnesses. Most of those costs are initiated by doctors like me. We're the ones who tell Mrs. Jones to come back for a follow-up visit in a month or send her for an X-ray or prescribe a medication. Costs are going up not because Mrs. Jones is old, or even sick—we're just providing more health care to her, and to her daughter and granddaughter too.

The problem with the aging population isn't that it will bankrupt us, but that we won't do it justice if we don't change the way we deliver health care services. Canadian medicare has traditionally been at its best in the hospital and in acute moments of crisis. But as the population ages, more Canadians will be living longer with chronic health conditions such as diabetes, high blood pressure, heart failure, and lung disease. These afflictions can dramatically reduce people's quality of life if they're not well managed in the community, including at home. And if people bounce in and out of hospital and the emergency department for every exacerbation of a chronic illness, they won't enjoy their old age. That really is unsustainable.

If, on the other hand, we can build a more robust and accessible system of home and community care, along with excellent primary care to support older people with chronic illness, we can welcome the demographic shift. The way we approach health care reform must, therefore, create new opportunities to treat patients with chronic disease, including seniors, outside the hospital.

The increases in health care spending we saw through the early 2000s have now slowed. If we can continue to be responsible about spending growth, we won't end up with the One Giant Ministry of Health that some people fear. The real question is whether the amount we spend is worth it. If health care spending is increasing and health outcomes are also getting better, that may be a good investment. But if health care spending is increasing and health outcomes aren't improving, then we have a problem.

On average, each year we spend about C$6000 per person on health care from public and private sources combined. (The United States averages nearly US$9000 annually per capita.) Of course, money spent on health care—whether public or private—is money that isn't available to spend on other things. How much do we want to spend on health care versus education, housing, food, or even entertainment and recreation?

If I told you that I'd bought a car for $6000, it probably wouldn't mean much unless I told you what kind of car. What make? What year? New or used? What we spend arguably matters less if we're getting good value for money.

It's hard to know whether our health care system is giving us good value for money because measuring the quality of a health care system is a complicated task. You can ask people how healthy they are. You can measure how long they live. You can look at how likely they are to die of diseases that we know medical science can cure. You can ask them how positive their last experience was with the system, or how long they had to wait for care. There is no single perfect measure, but if you look at a broad range of measures, including for vulnerable populations, and consider how much money you're spending, you can start to get a sense of the value for money spent. This is why it's so important to look at all three parts of the quality Triple Aim if you want to understand the performance of a health care system, and why so many international comparison studies don't tell the whole story.

———

The bottom line is that we don't have the worst health care outcomes in the world—but we don't have the best outcomes, either. And as we've seen, it isn't because we don't spend enough—we're one of the top ten spenders among forty-four peer countries.

What we spend in total, from both public and private sources, should be "enough." But we spend less *publicly* than many comparator nations, and particularly less in areas like prescription drugs, home care, mental health care, and dental care. Our system is less "public" than many people think (remember, only 70 percent of health care is financed with public dollars). We concentrate our spending on doctors and hospitals in order to maximize the advantages of single-payer health care: equity and administrative simplicity. Those are powerful reasons, but we could maintain that structure while increasing public funding of other services.

Rising costs are real, but what matters more than what we spend is what we get for it. Based on outcomes, our performance is solid—but too often, it's not excellent. We need to improve our performance in areas relating more to chronic, long-term problems as opposed to acute ones. And the Achilles heel of our system is access, especially with regard to long wait times for non-urgent, or planned, medical and surgical care.

If Canadians are as committed to medicare as we say we are, we must uphold the core values of our system. But we also want a set of improvements that will speed access to non-urgent care when we need it, control costs, and deliver better health for every dollar we spend. This means we must be prepared to make big and exciting changes.

What should those changes be? We could begin by discarding a bunch of bad ideas before we get to the good ones.

Health Care Zombies

Morris Barer and Bob Evans first coined the term "health care zombies" in 1998. A health care zombie is a terrible idea about health care that refuses to die. No matter how many times you drive an evidence-based stake through its heart, it rises from the (un)dead to confront you in the newspapers of the nation, ruining a perfectly good morning cup of coffee.

These ideas have often been proposed as solutions to the pressures on our health care system. But they've all been shown, time and time again, to weaken health care quality and sustainability. They also undermine our shared values.

User fees are a classic example. This zombie is resurrected year after year as a suggestion to deter inappropriate care and raise money. The idea behind user fees is that if people are required to pay either a fee (a copayment)—even a small one like $5 or $10—or a percentage of the total cost (co-insurance), they'll think twice before making an appointment for something "silly." They'll thus curb unnecessary use, and contribute some money out of pocket to help finance services. It's the "skin in the game" argument.

As an abundance of evidence shows, this is a bad idea for two reasons. First, user fees at the point of care indeed make patients think twice before seeking treatment. The problem is that these fees deter both unnecessary *and* necessary care. One U.S. study looked at how employees reacted when their employers switched them from a full-coverage plan to a high-deductible plan, in which employees had to pay a large sum out of pocket before their insurance kicked in. The employer saved money on the order of 15 percent, but the employees reduced the number of services they received to cut their own costs by much more: around 40 percent. They didn't shop around for better deals. Instead, all they did was get less care, risking their health or the health of their loved ones to save money.

This has been confirmed right here in Canada, in the birthplace of medicare. In the late 1960s the Saskatchewan government authorized physicians to charge patients $1.50 per clinic visit and $2.00 for outpatient services, including home, emergency, and hospital outpatient visits. The result was a drop in the use of those services—a drop most marked among people who could least afford to pay for health care and yet likely needed it most.

Do we really want a woman to think twice before coming in for her Pap test? Or a patient with chronic heart failure to put off her appointment with her cardiologist because she's already spent this month's income on other priorities? Do we want to burden parents with deciding whether their child's sudden stiff neck and cranky mood is due to a bad pillow or to meningitis? Especially among lower income people, user fees reduce usage of the kind of health care we want people to get. And in most cases, seeking reassurance from a health care provider doesn't constitute "abuse" of the system.

User fees are very blunt instruments for controlling usage. Beyond the human tragedies of these missed opportunities, care for advanced-stage illness is usually more expensive than the savings experienced by deterring preventive care. User fees are, as the saying goes, penny-wise and pound-foolish.

Second, user fees are a bad idea because they don't actually raise much money. If you set a user fee low enough to be affordable for everyone, it has to be pretty low. By the time you pay the administrators who have to collect and account for the copayments and co-insurance, you've created a costly bureaucracy that charges patients in order to support itself. In 2010, the Government of Quebec made waves by suggesting a "new" approach to dealing with increasing health care costs: a fee of $25 charged to the patient for every visit to a physician, to be paid in a lump sum at the end of the year when tax time rolled around. (Very low income people would not have to pay the fee.) Careful analysis of the proposal showed that it would fail to produce significant revenues for government. In order to raise enough money to make them "worth" the bureaucratic effort, user fees need to be pretty high. And once you start setting fees at the level needed to really raise revenue, you begin to block access for those with low incomes who may be quite sick. Alternatively, a significant part of the population would need to be exempted. So few people would be able to pay high fees that the policy would not generate considerable revenue.

———

In the parade of the undead, close behind the user-fee zombie we can usually find the private-pay zombie. The myth is that allowing wealthy patients to jump the queue will "take pressure off the public system."

I understand why this argument is intuitive. One might think that pulling one person out of the public queue would make the queue that much shorter, so that the private-pay tier functions as a safety valve of sorts for the public system. It's not true.

A study was conducted in Australia before and after that country moved from single-tier publicly funded care to two tiers, allowing privately funded care. It found that in those parts of the country that had more privately funded care, waits in the public system became *longer*. We saw the same results here in Canada when Manitoba experimented briefly with parallel private funding for cataract surgery, only to return to a fully public system when public wait lists got longer rather than shorter.

Why is this the case? Because the doctors, nurses, and others providing care in a privately funded system have to come from somewhere.

What people forget is that when a patient jumps the queue, a physician does too. The physician isn't available to treat the next person in the public queue, because she's busy treating the patient who just paid privately to jump that queue. The drain on the public system by providers exiting to the privately funded sector creates longer waiting lists in public health care.

In theory you could train enough doctors to staff both. But a health care system isn't just made up of doctors. You need nurses, nurse practitioners, physiotherapists, technologists, and an alphabet soup of other health care professionals. You need qualified administrators. You need a regulatory system to ensure quality and inspectors and accreditors to monitor it. Imagine the cost and time required to train the people and build the private tier in a way that wouldn't siphon resources from the public tier.

And in practice, a privately funded tier even provides an *incentive* to make wait times in the public system longer. A colleague once told me that in New Zealand, surgeons talk about "farming" in their practices: tilling the soil by keeping their public wait times long and then harvesting the benefits of high-paying patients in their private practices.

In 2006, the Canadian Medical Association reviewed all the evidence about two-tier and single-tier systems. Its report concluded that private health insurance does not improve access to services in the public system. It also concluded that private insurance does not lower costs or improve quality in the public system. In other words, access may improve for the small minority who can afford to pay; but patients in the public system can't expect anything good to happen for them if some people exit to a private tier.

———

So private financing won't reduce wait times for everyone, or help improve quality in our public system. Next in line comes the zombie of for-profit delivery. A clinic or hospital or facility might be owned by a group of investors rather than a couple of doctors, and those facilities have an obligation to bring profit back to their shareholders. Does it matter who delivers the service if the patient isn't being asked to pay out of pocket for it? Some argue that as long as patients use their health cards to pay for the service, it shouldn't matter whether those services are delivered by for-profit (more often called "private") clinics.

It does matter. As we move more services out of hospital and into the community, the number of private clinics inside the public system is growing. There are ardent supporters of such clinics, who believe that because they're driven by profit they'll be more efficient in their service delivery models.

But if we're to embrace for-profit hospitals and clinics in Canada, the quality of care has to be at least as good as it is in not-for-profit hospitals and clinics. And so far, that doesn't seem to be the case.

Instead, the evidence on for-profit hospitals, clinics, and long-term care facilities suggests that the care provided in them is inferior. In the United States, being admitted to a for-profit hospital instead of a not-for-profit hospital is associated with a statistically significant higher risk of dying. Having dialysis in a for-profit instead of a not-for-profit facility is also associated with an increased risk of death, even if the care is still publicly funded.

The evidence here in Canada points in the same direction. For example, a 2015 study looked at the rates of hospitalization and death among fifty thousand people newly admitted to Ontario long-term care homes (also known as nursing homes). Six months following admission, patients in for-profit homes were 16 percent more likely to have died, and almost 36 percent more likely to have been hospitalized, than those in not-for-profit homes.

Even if we figure out a way to regulate quality in for-profit facilities, the business models of the for-profit sector often involve upselling services and products that patients have to pay for. I think of my husband's friend who needed a colonoscopy, a service that was medically necessary and covered by OHIP. He was referred by his family doctor to a specialist who had hospital privileges but also worked in an out-of-hospital for-profit clinic. He was quoted a price and advised that he could jump the hospital queue and have the colonoscopy done in the private clinic a number of months earlier. It wasn't urgent, so he chose to wait for an opening in the hospital. He was subsequently contacted by the specialist's office and offered an appointment for the colonoscopy in the private clinic, but when he raised the question of fees, he was told that the procedure would be covered by OHIP. When he arrived he was seen by a dietitian, who counselled him on the importance of a high-fibre diet for his bowel health. He then had the procedure. On his way out the door, sedated, he was handed a bill for $300—the cost of the non-insured dietitian consultation that he'd never requested.

From orthopaedic surgery centres to colonoscopy clinics to boutique primary care offices, too many of these clinics find some way to charge patients for something. The core service is covered by taxpapers, but people leave having been upsold—whether it's a fancier lens when they get their cataract removed, or some sort of assessment that's only marginally related to the issue at hand. And in many cases, they aren't clearly offered the option *not* to pay for those extras, meaning that the for-profit delivery model ends up leading to compulsory private payment. So I remain unconvinced by claims that for-profit delivery can be incorporated into the Canadian health care system in ways that will help us achieve the Triple Aim of better health and a better patient experience at lower cost. Maybe it's possible, but I haven't yet seen the proof.

———

The zombies of user fees, private pay, and for-profit clinics all converge in one of the worst zombies of them all: the "Look at Europe" argument. European nations have models of health care that incorporate some aspects of private payment and for-profit medicine, say the supporters of this argument. Of course we don't want American-style health care, they concede, but why are we so afraid to follow the European model?

There is no such thing as the "European model" of health care. Each country in Europe has its own set of health and social services that have evolved in a very particular cultural, historical, and economic context.

Most European nations invest more public money in their health care systems than we do. They also tend to have much broader coverage and more generous social safety nets, and the higher tax rates to support them. Proponents of the so-called European model don't seem to argue for European tax rates or European child care policies, though. They pick the one thing they like about the French or the German or the Italian system and talk only about that specific policy, as if it existed in isolation. But we can't import French user fees and claim to have a French health care system any more than you can throw a Big Mac patty into a baguette and call it French cuisine.

In France, having private insurance does not let you jump the queue. It's voluntary and used primarily to cover the copayments charged in the public system. And, owing to concerns about fairness, regulations are increasingly aimed at preventing physicians from charging more money privately than they do publicly.

In Germany, only 10 percent of the population has private health insurance, and those who do must leave the publicly funded system entirely. I think it's unlikely that Canadians would be interested in such a model.

Another important consideration when comparing Canada to Europe is the border we share with the United States. Canadian doctors earn more money than doctors in many European countries—and one of the market forces that drive the price of physician labour in Canada is the fact that we're in competition with the United States for our health care workforce. It's something that France, for example, doesn't really have to contend with.

That shared border has another important effect. Our trade agreements with the United States, including NAFTA, contain clauses that preserve the ability of Canadian governments to maintain single-tier medicare by regulating private investment in the health care sector, including by American firms. But if we were to move to private payment and for-profit delivery, medicare would no longer have those protections. We can't switch to "European style" health care and not end up with American health care corporations surging into our system. To claim that we could is to fundamentally misunderstand our political, economic, and geographic reality.

The suggestion that a magical "European model" will solve all our problems usually stems from a desire to allow some people to pay privately to jump the queue and some doctors to charge more for their services. It's nearly always made with a dogmatic belief in the "free market," despite all the evidence of its inefficiency in the health care sector.

That said, it's always worth learning how other countries organize their services so that we might improve care in our own. In many European countries, for example, home and community care are much better integrated with other health and social services. We can certainly take the best of those care delivery models and adapt them for the Canadian context.

———

When I asked my mother to write down her parents' story for me to include in this book, she finished her message with a reference to the Canada Health Act. "We rejoiced when Monique Bégin and the federal government of the day passed the Canada Health Act in 1984," she wrote. "It was far too late for our family, but it signalled the dawn of new hope for all Canadians."

Many Canadians who remember life before medicare still feel this way. But in the context of an aging population, new technologies, increasing utilization of services of questionable value, and concerns about system sustainability, medicare needs new approaches.

Having dispensed with the zombies, let's explore those new approaches. In this book, with gratitude to the innovators who think about how to improve our system, I'm pulling together the six Big Ideas

I believe can best improve the health of Canadians. They aren't my ideas. But they're well formulated, they're grounded in good evidence, and they meet the two tests for delivering on the promise of medicare. They would improve the Triple Aim of our health care system, delivering accessible, high-quality services in an equitable way. And they're worthy of an iconic program.

These Big Ideas would help us get better—much better. Now. And each idea is dedicated to a particular Canadian patient, because it's important to remember who we're in this for.

BIG IDEA 1

ABIDA: THE RETURN
TO RELATIONSHIPS

Primary Care:
When It Works, It Works

When I first met Abida, I was assuming her care from the family doctor whose practice I took over at Women's College Hospital in 2006. My office is part of the Family Practice Health Centre at the hospital, a large clinic that I was excited to join just six months into my first year of practice.

Even then, in her early sixties, Abida was already what we call a "complex patient," a woman with many medical problems. She had at least four specialist physicians in her life—a cardiologist, a gastroenterologist, an endocrinologist, and a surgeon who had operated on her years before but continued to see her annually—and at least two teams of physical therapists, dietitians, and other professionals who helped her manage her osteoporosis and poor mobility.

Each of these people took excellent care of the body part they were responsible for. But frankly, none of them could take care of Abida.

Abida is originally from Bangladesh, and immigrated to Canada when she was already married. Two of her four sons were born in Canada. Her marriage was arranged, and unlike some of my patients whose arranged marriages are happy ones, she felt trapped in it. Her husband is a controlling and negative person. Abida never worked outside the home and has no path to financial independence. When her children grew up and left the house, her husband became even more controlling: she couldn't get access to enough money to get her hair done unless she managed to catch him in a "generous" mood; she would cook all day only to have him insult the food she put in front of him at the dinner table. She felt isolated and humiliated, but she had, as she put it, "nowhere to go."

At the time we met, Abida's body knew that her situation was dire, and it had started to manifest the effects. She had chest pain. Palpitations. Dizziness. A constant low-grade headache. Memory loss. Hip pain. Trouble with her balance. The list of vague, but very real, physical symptoms was long and growing. Often she would tell one of her skilled and dedicated specialists about her headaches or belly upset, which would inevitably lead to referral to another specialist who dealt with that body part. Other times she would come to our clinic and see the evening doctor on call about weakness or chest pain. He or she would look at her long list of medical problems and worry about the worst— stroke, heart attack—and then send her to the emergency department, where Abida would inevitably spend the night being carefully investigated and observed.

Her problems were not "in her head." As she aged, she accumulated more and more significant medical problems, including chronic lung disease, bowel troubles, and a series of mini-strokes. But just as often there would be no identifiable cause for her distress, and after a night in the emergency department or a few days in hospital, she'd be sent home with more specialist follow-up. She was rapidly becoming a full-time patient.

I have now been Abida's family doctor for more than ten years. She's one of the many patients who've helped me grow into a more mature physician, sometimes through trial and painful error. We've learned together how her physical symptoms worsen when things are especially difficult at home. We've developed safety plans in case her husband becomes physically violent, and discussed many times the possibility that she might leave him—something I suspect she will never do. We've slowly reduced the number of medications she takes and the number of specialists she sees. Instead, she sees me more frequently than she used to—weekly, if necessary—and she's developed a close relationship with the terrific nurse on my team, who is her first point of contact for a phone call about a twisted ankle or a question about her medications. We've tried to limit the number of times she gets sent to the emergency department by ensuring that she sees me, rather than another provider, as much as possible. Because I know her, I'm better able to judge whether a symptom represents a substantial change.

Often she comes with a list of physical concerns and I just sit and listen, empathizing with how difficult or annoying or frustrating a symptom must be without ordering any tests or recommending any particular treatment. In recent years I've learned to focus on supporting anything she can do to improve her social life and interactions, encouraging her to spend time out of the house and get more involved in her spiritual community. I've helped her manage her many medical illnesses as best I can, and if I need help from a specialist I increasingly try to phone or email one for advice rather than sending her off for an appointment that will inevitably lead to more tests and interventions. The more I know Abida, and the better I understand my role, it seems the less I "do" to her. I've slowly learned how to be there for her without always trying to fix her.

As all this has gone on, we've developed a bond. She's watched my career develop, sometimes coming in to tell me that she saw me on the news talking about vaccinations or healthy eating and thought I did a good job. In 2009 she witnessed my growing belly and dropped off a small gift when my daughter was born. She asks advice not only about her own health, but the health of her husband and sons. In other words, we have a relationship. And there is no doubt in my mind that as imperfect as I am, my involvement in her care over time has decreased her physical risks and improved her overall health, while saving the health care system money.

———

When I was a medical student, I loved the rotations through the wards of local hospitals in London, Ontario. During my surgical month I experienced the immense satisfaction of helping to remove a tumour growth and "fixing" the patient, so I wanted to be a surgeon. When I watched what a dignified death can look like on the palliative care ward, I wanted to do palliative care. As I felt with a shaking hand the unstoppable force of a baby being born, I wanted to be an obstetrician. In every rotation, I was encouraged by terrific mentors to join their specialty, and the refrain was consistent: "You're too smart to be a family doctor."

I'm so glad I didn't listen.

I have the best job on earth. At the beginning of every clinic, I look over my list of patients. That fifty-six-year-old woman booked at ten-fifteen might be coming in for a blood pressure check. Or maybe she has a tumour compressing her spinal cord and will need to be shipped out of my office immediately by ambulance. She may need an abscess drained. Or her kids are getting into serious trouble with the law. Perhaps she's finally ready to talk about the three generous servings of vodka she drinks most nights of the week. Or she's been coughing up blood and is terrified she has lung cancer just as her mother did. My mind has to be open to every possibility in the wide world of medicine.

The magic of family medicine does not lie only in the range of diagnostic and therapeutic work. When we teach residents to be family doctors, we tell them that *"In hospitals, the diseases stay and the people come and go; in general practice, the people stay and the diseases come and go."* The disease coming in this afternoon may be a surprise to me, but the person isn't. I know Abida, and she knows me. Maybe we shared a profound moment the last time she came in, when she told me about the history of abuse in her family, or her fear of developing dementia. She always comments on my shoes. We have connected on issues mundane and profound. There are things she'll tell me that she wouldn't tell anyone else, and because of that, while we aren't friends, I hold her in my heart.

Good primary care requires a broad knowledge base. It also requires humility, the ability to sit with the discomfort of uncertainty and help patients do the same, a profound respect for the role of specialists, and a deep confidence that a health care provider who knows the person is at least as important to her health as one who specializes in the disease.

And when it's well organized and supported, a primary care practice does much more than just take care of the individuals who come through the door. It serves as a connecting point for the entirety of a person's journey through the health care system, and it reaches beyond its walls to improve the health of the community it serves. A provider or group of providers can identify a population for whose health they are responsible and track that population using data, reaching out to engage in prevention and screening efforts. They can monitor and support patients with chronic diseases, and function as the hub for health and social services in the community.

When it works, it really works. That's the Big Idea in this section: relationship-based primary care for every Canadian. This means that every individual should have a relationship with a primary care doctor or nurse practitioner. It also means that every primary care group should have good relationships with the rest of the health care system, and with the community in which all are embedded.

———

In a society that fetishizes specialization and dramatic, life-saving measures, the value of generalism can be overlooked or minimized. This isn't just a Canadian phenomenon. From the United Kingdom to India to the United States, primary care is critically important and yet, paradoxically, often undervalued. There are lots of reasons for this, but one is that as medical technology advances, it can be hard for people to remember that treatment from specialists isn't always better than treatment from generalists. For many kinds of care, including prevention, screening, and the management of chronic disease, treatment from a generalist who knows you is nearly always your best bet. Relationship-based care from a generalist can and should be holistic: as British general practitioner and medical leader Dr. Iona Heath has said, *"A death from a non-cardiac cause can be regarded as a triumph for a cardiologist, but all deaths fall within the remit of the GP."*

Primary care is also critical to ensuring that our health care system will be sustainable. Systems that focus on good primary care are more cost-effective, more equitable, and deliver higher quality care overall.

A big part of the reason for this is that primary care is the best place to help people manage chronic disease. As medical science has enabled an increasing number of people to survive previously fatal problems like cardiovascular disease and cancers, people are living longer and developing more chronic conditions like high blood pressure, diabetes, and heart and lung disease. To have each of these diseases treated by a different specialist, as Abida was doing when I met her, is not only time-consuming and confusing for the patient but expensive for the system.

In the absence of primary care from a trusted provider, the rest of the system picks up the slack—at much higher cost. Consider one study that looked at men who were seen in a hospital emergency room with severe, uncontrolled high blood pressure, a condition that can lead to stroke and kidney failure, among other complications. Nearly all these patients had previously been diagnosed with high blood pressure, knew they had it, and had been prescribed medications. But severe, uncontrolled high blood pressure was found to be more than four times more common among patients who did not have their own primary care doctor. Study after study has confirmed that when a patient doesn't have a family doctor, both the patient and the rest of the system suffer. Dr. Lesley Barron, a Canadian surgeon who writes a thoughtful blog, put it this way:

A man was referred to me by a hospital emergency department (ED). He presented there on a Friday night with a complaint. For those of you who are fortunate enough to have never needed to use an emergency room, weekend evenings are the worst time to have to use an ED. Now all the people who don't have a family doctor, PLUS all the people who do have one but they aren't open, PLUS all the people who are too sick to go to their family doctor or have been to their GPs already and been sent on to the hospital, are there waiting to be assessed and treated. . . . So this guy shows up on a Friday night and waits. And waits. And waits some more. He is seen, discharged, and a referral sent to me to ask for an assessment of his condition, which I do in a few days. I'm not going to say what his condition was, but it was not life threatening, nor was was it surgical, and [it] did not require any management or testing other than reassurance that nothing was going on here. After I assessed him, I asked for the name of his family doctor, to send a note so they are kept informed as to what is going on with him. . . . "I'm healthy," he promptly replied. "I don't need a family doctor." I looked at him. I didn't get mad, but it was a little frustrating. "You just PROVED you need a family doctor," I said. "You had to go to an ED on a Friday night to get a referral for something that could have been easily dealt with by a family doctor." He looked a little sheepish. I offered to refer him on to a GP colleague who was accepting new patients—an offer he accepted. I understand a lot of other conditions have now been uncovered and are being treated in this fellow. . . .

Most people are not going to be healthy their entire lives and then drop dead. It's just not done that way anymore. Let's say you develop some symptoms, possibly related to mental illness. Do you really want to be going for diagnosis, treatment and follow-up in an ED or a walk-in clinic? It is safer, faster, cheaper and better care to be assessed by someone who knows you, and/or has your file to refer back to. . . .

The notion of being seen by "someone who knows you" is central to primary care. The best place to integrate all your health needs is a place where, like the bar in *Cheers*, everybody knows your name.

In an ideal world you shouldn't need to see your family doctor often. But in the real world, we all develop concerns sooner or later. Many more Canadians have contact with the primary care system than they ever see a specialist or stay in a hospital. More than two hundred Canadian adults out of every thousand will contact their family physician in a given month, but only seventy will have contact with a specialist and even fewer will be hospitalized: eight Canadians per thousand. High-performing health care systems all over the world are built on a strong foundation of primary care.

Even more Canadians have chronic conditions but don't interact much with the health care system at all. These are the people for whom good care outside the hospital can make a real difference.

Every Canadian should have someone whom they view as their "personal provider," usually a family doctor or a nurse practitioner. We're most of the way there: approximately 85 percent of Canadians report that they have a family physician, a proportion that rises to 95 percent for adults with multiple chronic illnesses. Moreover, Canadians tend to rate their primary care experiences very highly, once they're able to get in the door. For example, we know that nearly three-quarters of those surveyed in 2013 rated the care they received in their regular doctor's office as "very good" or "excellent." But to achieve the full potential of relationship-based primary care, we have a lot more work to do.

I focus on family medicine because the vast majority of primary care in Canada is delivered by family doctors, and that's likely to continue to be the case. Having said that, primary care is not the sole remit of doctors. Nurses, nurse practitioners, physician assistants, midwives, pharmacists, social workers, dietitians, and a wide range of other providers are increasingly the first point of contact with the health care system. In some communities, people receive nearly all their primary care from nurses with advanced training. And in remote communities throughout Canada's vast north, where there are very few physicians or nurse practitioners, they may receive their primary care from community health workers.

There is no magic to an MD degree that makes a doctor the only person suitable for providing high-quality primary care. Other providers play important roles in disease prevention, health promotion, and the treatment of illness. In the case of primary care nurse practitioners, their training enables them to perform work formerly thought of as "doctor" work.

I'm not worried that a nurse practitioner or any other provider might do much (or even all) of what I do as a family physician. They're well-trained and capable, and when they bump up against the limits of their expertise, they bring a doctor into the mix—just as I seek other expertise when I hit my own limits. Frankly, there is more than enough work to go around.

What matters to me isn't who does the work, but that the work drives primary care to live up to its potential. This means that we can't just look to download tasks onto less costly providers at the expense of relationships, or add more providers to the team without a clear purpose and good evidence that their participation improves the health of the community, improves the patient's experience of care, and saves the system money—the Triple Aim. As a doctor and a citizen I want to know that every primary care provider is prepared to commit to three critical relationships: with patients, with the other parts of the health care system, and with the broader population they serve.

Three Relationships for Health

The way family physicians think about their work may surprise you. When people ask me what kind of medicine I practise, the answer "I'm a family doctor" is usually met with one of two responses: either "Are you taking patients?" or "Are you planning to specialize in something?" Of course, I do specialize in something, but it isn't a body part. Family doctors specialize in relationships.

Before family medicine became a recognized specialty in Canada in the early 1990s, doctors could do a one-year rotating internship after medical school and hang a shingle as a "general practitioner," or GP. Today, family medicine in Canada requires a two-year residency program after the completion of a medical degree. At the end of that training, graduates are specialists in generalism.

Family physicians are trained in recognizing undifferentiated disease and managing uncertainty. As you probably noticed the last time you had an appointment with your doctor or nurse practitioner, primary care is a low-tech environment. Part of the reason why it's so much less expensive than hospital-based care is that the care is usually one on one, and there are very few of those "machines that go ping" that we see in hospitals. Yet despite the fact that the tools we use are mostly our eyes, ears, and brains, family doctors are usually responsible for making the initial diagnosis upon which subsequent care is based. The importance of the accuracy of that initial diagnosis cannot be overstated. Dr. Iona Heath, the U.K. primary care leader mentioned earlier, has said that it requires us to combine "a robust appreciation of the range of the normal with a high index of suspicion for the dangerous."

One of the most important things we do in primary care is what Dr. Heath has called "patrolling the border" between illness and disease.

Disease is what we learn about in medical-school textbooks: a somewhat arbitrary set of definitions that have developed over time based on pattern recognition. "Angina" and "schizophrenia" are just shorthand ways to refer to a set of symptoms and signs that tend to occur together.

Illness, on the other hand, is an individual human being's experience of being unwell. It is "a perception of something being wrong, a sense of unease in the functioning of the body or mind." Since no two people are the same, no two people have the same experience of illness, even if they share the same disease label.

Primary care providers like family doctors see more illness than disease—we spend much of our time accompanying patients along the journey of their experience of feeling unwell, whether they have acquired a disease label or not.

Therefore, one of the important functions of primary care is to allow our patients to experience illness without over-interpreting, over-labelling, or overtreating them. Much illness resolves on its own, so that one of the great skills of family medicine is the appropriate use of *time*—giving the body a chance to heal itself without missing the moments when more intervention is needed.

As a result of our work patrolling this boundary, family physicians are medical experts in the management of uncertainty. And we address uncertainty in myriad ways, including providing patients with objectivity, knowledge, and companionship.

How do we hold the border between illness and disease, or help our patients cope with uncertainty about the future? The most important principle that we teach our residents in family medicine training is that *the patient–physician relationship is central to the role of the family physician.* The secret sauce of primary care is the relationship.

Abida and I have learned together about the power of the relationship in patrolling the border between illness and disease. Because we know each other well, when she reports discomfort in her foot, for example, I listen and then I examine her. If I don't see anything of concern, I can then say, "I'm not sure what might be causing that, but it doesn't sound sinister to me. Let's wait and see whether it goes away on its own rather than sending you for X-rays or blood tests today. We can reassess it in two weeks. In the meantime, try ice and heat to see if that will help with the pain." I don't doubt that her foot hurts, but I don't jump to label her with a disease. It's because of the trust she has in me, earned over these many years, that she feels comfortable waiting as I suggest—and it's because I've come to know her as well as I do that I feel reasonably certain it's safe to do so. For Abida, this is critical, because so often her symptoms are vague and could lead to enormous over-investigation if we did not hold that boundary.

Specialists also develop relationships with their patients, sometimes over many years. But family practice as a discipline explicitly defines itself by that relationship. Dr. Ian McWhinney, one of the founders of modern family medicine, articulated this beautifully when he said that in family medicine, "the relationship is usually prior to content. We know people before we know what their illnesses will be."

In family medicine we teach our residents that every interaction with a patient, whether it's to discuss a disintegrating marriage or a wart on the sole of the foot, must be seen as an opportunity to strengthen the relationship. I think of these as little deposits in a "relationship bank," an account that accrues interest over time.

If we're successful, people will feel heard and seen, and will have an enhanced ability to take care of their own health. They will need less time in our office, or anyone else's for that matter, and they will forgive us our bad days, insensitive moments, and (true story) that time we forgot to cancel their clinic appointment before taking a long birthday weekend away.

It is this relationship that almost certainly underpins the repeated observation that health care systems centred on primary care are less expensive than those that are not. People who trust in and get good care from their family physician will need specialty care and hospital care less often. This is not just because of the "gatekeeper" function of primary care, in which a referral is needed to see a specialist; it's because in going to see their family doctors, patients' concerns may be addressed and no further interaction with the health care system may be needed.

I have experienced this with Abida. Over the years that we've worked together on her health, she's stopped going to the emergency department so frequently. She has fewer specialists involved in her care, and when she does see specialists, she usually comes back to me to ask my views about the investigations or treatments they've recommended. This isn't because she doesn't trust the experts; it's because she knows that I know the whole of her story and can put their recommendations into her life's context for her.

The effectiveness of our interaction depends on mutual respect as much as it does on content expertise. Without trust and a relationship, family doctors are at risk of becoming referral and prescription machines. And without ready access to one's trusted family doctor, a patient is at risk of becoming unmoored in the health care system.

———

Now I'm going to say something controversial: some kinds of health care don't require a deep relationship. In fact, for many kinds of specialty services—including surgery—experience has shown that we can reduce wait times and improve experience by having less, not more, "face time" with specialists, or with one particular specialist. Team-based care, where much of the pre- and post-procedure work is done by non-physician providers, and models where people are seen by the next available team member rather than waiting for a particular doctor have shown great promise in many parts of the health care system.

This doesn't hold true across the board, of course. In some kinds of specialty services, relationships are critical. (Examples like psychiatry and palliative care leap to mind.) But sometimes relationships can be built with a team or even an organization rather than with an individual specialist. Trust that the service is high quality and reliable may not depend on a deep and ongoing relationship with a single health care provider.

In primary care, however, the ongoing relationship is the core of our ability to be effective.

This is why I struggle with walk-in clinics. I understand why they exist. It's convenient to just pop down during your lunch hour to the clinic in the basement of your office building. Or maybe you tried to make an appointment with your family doctor and she couldn't get you in for two weeks. But even most doctors who work in them, if they're really being honest, will tell you that a walk-in clinic isn't ideal primary care. There's no continuity, no comprehensive chart that can be used for your ongoing care, and usually no communication back to anyone who will ever see you again. The concept of relationship-based care generally goes out the window.

You might think that all you need is a quick prescription renewal or blood test requisition. That's a legitimate agenda. But if you'd seen your family doctor, he could have used that opportunity to compare your blood pressure to last time, causing him to notice that it's creeping up. He could have reminded you that you're due for a Pap smear in three months and asked you to book it on your way out. You might have backed into a conversation about your weight, causing you to consider bringing your lunch to work instead of eating that horrible stuff with gravy on it in the cafeteria. You could have connected, investing in the "relationship bank" that you may well need to withdraw from in the future.

In a perfect world we wouldn't need walk-in clinics, because all Canadians would be able to see their own personal primary care provider (or at least a team member who has access to their chart with their medical history) within a day or two if that's what they need. When Abida's lung disease flares and she starts to feel more short of breath, she needs to be seen now—not three days from now. I can't be personally available to her 24 hours a day, 365 days a year, and I don't think anyone expects that of me. But I can ensure that someone who has access to Abida's chart and can connect back with me will see her when she needs to be seen, by sharing responsibility with my colleagues. That means same-day appointments; evening, weekend, and holiday appointments; and someone on call who can answer Abida's questions about her breathing in the middle of the night.

It may be that in some communities the best answer will be to integrate walk-in clinics with the rest of the system, so that at least I get some notification when my patients have been seen elsewhere and can follow up with them. In other places, teams will establish walk-in options of their own so that patients who need to be seen urgently can drop in without an appointment and see a team member, if not their own doctor. To me, those options are preferable to a totally unconnected clinic that doesn't provide any continuity of care.

———

It's important to recognize the real value and importance of the primary care relationship, but we shouldn't romanticize it. Like every relationship, this one has its ups and downs. I'm bound to have an off day and say the wrong thing sometimes, especially when the waiting room is full and I had an argument with my spouse last night, or when the previous patient had to be sent to the hospital because she was suicidal. You'd be right to feel annoyed when you sense that I'm distracted or when I made you sit too long in the waiting room. And you're bound to push my own buttons sometimes, maybe by asking for a dermatologist referral to treat your mild acne or by refusing a tetanus vaccination for your child. We may not have chosen each other and maybe the perfect family doctor for you would be a different kind of person. But if you're in my practice, I'm committed to making it work—and my colleagues feel the same way.

It's a rare case that a family doctor "fires" a patient—I haven't done it, and most doctors feel it should only be done in really exceptional circumstances. I do have patients who've left my practice. In most cases I called them to ask why, or the nurse I work with did, so as to not put them on the spot. From their answers I learned things about myself and my practice, and usually I agreed that we weren't a good fit. I have many more patients who've stayed in my practice and we've made it work, even though we might not have chosen each other for compatibility if online matching existed for this sort of thing. There's something that happens when the door clicks shut in that exam room that makes us both want to try.

Like many relationships, neither of us may give it much of a second thought until one day when it suddenly matters a lot. I think about one patient whom I used to see only once every year or so. We had accumulated a fair number of moments together over the years, though many of them were focused on her daughter's health care needs rather than hers. Yet the cumulative effect of those small interactions was that we had invested in the relationship bank together. This meant that when her breast cancer was diagnosed—the same disease that killed her mother, so you can imagine her reaction—we had an established connection we could draw on. I believe it made a difference in my ability to give her what she needed, and for her to approach her treatment plan with dignity and optimism.

———

The relationship between a primary health care provider and her patient allows us to provide care that is personalized. But sometimes the flexibility of approaches that comes along with that can be a bad thing. Among the tensions family doctors have to grapple with is the one between our desire to provide personalized care and our duty to stick with guidelines for the care of people with particular conditions.

In general, health care is moving toward more standardized approaches to the treatment of many illnesses, and that's mostly good.

It's helped us make enormous improvements in some areas over the last two decades, such as screening for and treating high blood pressure. Whether it's making sure that everyone over fifty is offered colon cancer screening, giving diabetics a regular eye exam, or vaccinating people with chronic lung disease against pneumonia, there are some things that we know every person with a given disease needs. But we aren't yet doing a good enough job of making sure they get them. In managing chronic disease, then, it's critically important that primary care teams step up and start practising *consistently*.

Yet family doctors have sometimes pushed back against cookie-cutter approaches to disease management. This pushback comes in part from a good place. We have to manage the reality that giving people the care they "should get" for a particular disease and paying attention to the priority for that person at a given moment in time may not always be compatible. You might "need" to get your blood pressure down eight more points. But you might rather spend the time we have together talking about how to manage the stress in your job—and I might agree with you on that priority. Or we might decide to set aside the diabetes guidelines for now because you also have asthma and would prefer to focus on dealing with that.

One of the reasons why disease-based guidelines are often less useful in primary care is that they aren't developed by family doctors. Specialists are three times more likely to contribute to drafting guidelines than are family physicians, with the result that those guidelines often fail to reflect the realities of primary care.

Furthermore, as we age, we all accumulate diagnoses, so that the list of guidelines and checklists that applies to each of us just grows. When you add up the amount of time required for a primary care physician to provide the recommended preventive services to patients as well as the recommended manoeuvres for the ten most common chronic conditions, the average family doctor could spend between eleven and eighteen hours per day just delivering preventive and chronic illness care. This is before we see anyone with an acute problem, fill out a form, answer a phone call, or have breakfast.

When I think about the number of guidelines that could potentially apply to a patient like Abida, my mind goes numb. She has a diagnosis for nearly every body part. She has heart disease, lung disease, thyroid disease, high cholesterol, arthritis, and osteoporosis. There are, of course, full sets of practice guidelines for each of these problems. Abida is also older and becoming frailer, so she's at risk of falls, depression, social isolation, and a whole range of other problems—each of which I would love to address in a proactive way, and none of which may jell with *her* priorities, which often come back to needing a safe place to talk about what's happening at home. So there has to be a balance.

To me, guidelines are useful in pushing us to build more reliable and standardized systems for taking care of people. It matters that I follow the same routine, every time, for every prenatal visit for every pregnant woman, so that none of the important steps are missed—even if we decide together not to do some things that the guideline says we should. Just the process of having that conversation increases reliability, and if done right, deepens the relationship.

———

The doctor–patient relationship is the foundation of high-functioning primary care, but there are two other relationships that are also critical to achieving the Big Idea of relationship-based primary care for every Canadian.

One is the relationship of your doctor's office to the rest of the health care system. As a family doctor, I'm the go-to health resource for the group of people with whose care I'm tasked. My job isn't only to develop relationships with those patients and take care of them, but to be their point of entry to and exit from many other services.

To practise good primary care I need to understand how the local health care system works, and how to make it work for you. How does one get to see a specialist in the neighbourhood? Which hospital offers general neurology, and which just headache consultation? Which ear surgeon has the shortest wait time? Which one is efficient, but lacks bed-side manner? Which physiotherapist offers discounted rates for low-income people? How do I know when my patient has been admitted or discharged from a local hospital? By keeping up to date on the answers to these types of questions, I can effectively coordinate care for my patients.

This relationship with the system is updated and improved by my returning patients. They feel they can tell me where the waits are long or the service terrific. The team of health care providers I work with does the same. We constantly send each other quick messages to ask who knows a great chiropodist in the north end of the city, or how to get a psycho-educational assessment for a kid who's struggling in school.

These informal networks do the job, but a more organized system for referrals would be so welcome in my universe. I'd love to feel confident that I was sending each patient to a competent, caring provider (or team) who'll see them quickly, and I'd happily trade some of my informal con-nections for that reliability. But even when that day comes, the role of connector will still be a big part of my job.

In this role, primary care providers are medical experts in managing information. And there's a lot of it: specialist consultation advice, lab and medical imaging results, email messages, diagrams of different body parts, hospital discharge summaries, illegible pink sheets of paper that once made up the back page of an emergency department record in trip-licate—all must be integrated into a single chart that tells your medical story over time. We also manage a constantly shifting database of infor-mation about the system around us so that we can help you get the ser-vices you need.

The important relationship between primary care and the rest of the system doesn't always work well. And when I run up against the brick wall of some other silo in the health care system that prevents me from getting what I feel a patient needs, I get mad. Luckily, the twenty-first century offers a productive outlet for professional frustration: the com-plaint email. Here are two (paraphrased, and admittedly rather testy) emails I've sent to one hospital's CEO and another hospital's VP in downtown Toronto over the last couple of years. I share them because I think they illustrate what happens when the relationship between primary care and the rest of the system breaks down—which fortunately isn't all the time.

September 2010

Dear [Hospital CEO],

Are you aware that when a patient dies in your hospital, no one informs their family doctor?

I learned about this unbelievable oversight this week, when our clinic staff called a 54-year-old woman in my practice to inform her she is due for a pap smear. Her son, who answered the phone, informed the secretary that she had a sudden cardiac arrest three months ago. She was rushed to your organization by ambulance, spent two weeks in your ICU, and subsequently passed away.

I'm sure you can appreciate how upsetting it was for the son to have to explain this to his own family physician's office. How is it possible that you have no process for informing the primary care providers of patients in your organization that our patients are deceased?

September 2015

Hi [Hospital VP],

I'm writing to give you feedback about an experience I had with your hospital this week as a primary care provider in the neighbourhood.

I saw a patient Wednesday evening in my clinic who had features suggestive of a possible neurosurgical emergency. The case was a tricky one with grey areas, and I was uncertain how best to help her get assessed rapidly, whether she needed to be assessed immediately, and whether there was more that needed to be done for her in the short term.

I paged neurosurgery on call at your hospital to ask their advice about how to manage the case. I was on the phone for 45 minutes, running progressively more late with the other patients sitting in the waiting room. At one point Dr. [XX], the surgeon on call, was patched in to the call but when the nurse who was holding the phone for me asked him to hold while she ran to get me, he hung up. When I called back he refused to take my phone call. The hospital operator told me to call 911, which was exactly what I had been trying to avoid.

We did call 911. My 74-year-old patient, who was in excruciating pain, sat in your emergency department until 1:30 in the morning and was eventually seen by the ED doc, had some imaging, and was sent home and told to come back to me to be referred as an outpatient to the various specialists she should see.

I'm sure you can imagine that this outcome was upsetting for my patient, and also for me. I'm not sure why I should stay in clinic until 8 pm seeing patients to give them rapid and convenient access to primary care if the purpose is not to keep them out of the ED. I can't do that effectively without specialist backup when I run up against the limits of my scope of practice or my expertise. . . .

Much as I was frustrated with Dr. [XX] that night, I suspect the response may have been similar if I had called any number of doctors. The family doc is dependent on the mercy of the individual at the other end of the line to help us figure out how to navigate the system, instead of feeling backed up by a community of health care workers who want to help us do our best for people.

I understand these are big issues to grapple with and that in general, hospital culture has been one of dealing with those people who are already present in the building, and not worrying much about the primary care community. But when I practised in rural northern Ontario, the specialists in [YY] hospital understood very clearly that their role was to be a resource to anyone in the catchment area who needed them. Through the use of telephone specialist backup, we managed dozens of cases both in clinic and in the ED that otherwise would have had to be transferred to the big hospital 300 km away.

In each of these cases, the hospital administrator responded quickly and appropriately. But as you can no doubt tell from the tone of my emails, the disconnect between the primary care universe and the hospital universe is an ongoing source of difficulty for patients and irritation for providers. Indeed, the fact that we regard each as living in a separate universe is part of the problem.

That disconnect isn't just on the hospital side. My specialist friends tell me about the patients who come to their offices with virtually no information about the referral request from the family doctor, forcing these specialists to start from scratch and repeat investigations they know have already been done, wasting time and money in the process. Emergency department doctors and nurses experience extreme frustration when patients show up because their family doctor went on vacation and simply turned on the answering machine for two weeks, leaving people with no choice but to go to the ED or a walk-in clinic. And friends have shared stories of family physicians who refer their patients to specialists so freely that they feel it would be easier just to go see a specialist directly for any concern. This isn't relationship-based primary care. We can do better.

That said, when the relationship between primary care and the rest of the system works well, the results can be extraordinary. I was in clinic recently when the secretary pulled me out of an exam room to take a phone call from a pediatrician at a local hospital. She was calling to tell me that one of my patients had been admitted with a potentially dangerous problem. She wanted me to know so that when he was discharged I could see him quickly and follow him closely—and she wanted to share some recommendations for monitoring him over time. It took about three minutes, and it wasn't a fancy or high-tech integration solution. It was just a human interaction by telephone. But it saved me—and the patient and his parents—a lot of work trying to piece together exactly what had been done in hospital and what my role needed to be.

More systematic efforts are being made to ensure consistently good communication between primary care and hospitals. If you live in British

Columbia, for example, your family doctor now has access to a program called RACE—Rapid Access to Consultative Expertise. This is a telephone advice line that family doctors can call to speak with a specialist for advice about patient care. Phone calls are directly routed to a specialist's cell phone or pager. An evaluation of the program revealed that 80 percent of calls were answered within ten minutes and that nearly one-third of calls prevented an emergency department visit. This and other initiatives across the country give me hope for the future of the primary care–health system relationship.

And these kinds of initiatives are exactly what I need to be able to take good care of someone like Abida. Because of her medical and social complexity, when a specialist meets Abida for the first time she often ends up with more investigations that she may or may not follow through on. When I'm able to get a specialist on the phone instead, he or she can often talk me through Abida's options so that she and I can then work together on a plan tailored to her needs. This also saves Abida the time and irritation of having to tell her story to someone new all over again.

———

The other relationship that's critical for high-functioning primary care is the one where we have the most work to do: the one between primary care providers and the population we serve.

We're only just beginning to consider the concept of "managing the health of a population" in Canadian primary care. That population would usually be a geographic one, though not always: some practices may specifically serve people living with HIV or adults with developmental disabilities who travel significant distances to see primary care providers with special expertise. But most of the time a primary care practice should serve the people who live or work in a given neighbourhood or community, no matter what their diagnoses. This has long been a stated principle in Canadian primary care, and is the approach taken in high-performing health systems: rather than waiting for patients to show up on the doorstep, doctors and teams who practise primary care see it as their job to improve the health of the people in their neighbourhood.

Since the advent of electronic medical records, our ability to do that job has been transformed. When I started out I had no way of knowing, say, who the diabetics in my practice were unless they came in the door. Now, with just a few keystrokes, my electronic record provides me with a list of everyone with that diagnosis, when they were last seen, and whether they're due for routine diabetes testing and care. This allows me to reach out to people proactively and ask them to get their eyes checked or have their blood sugar tested.

Developing a relationship with my practice population means that, rather than waiting for people to call for an appointment, I need to establish routine ways of reminding families when it's time for children's immunizations or women's Pap smears. It also means that I should track how many frail elderly patients are in my practice and organize home visits and non-medical support services for them. One day soon it will mean that, when one of my patients is discharged from a local hospital, I'll be automatically notified by email and my office will reach out to that person to book a follow-up appointment so that we can debrief together.

Every primary care practice needs to use an electronic medical record, and we're getting there: today about three-quarters of primary care doctors in Canada use them—a proportion that has nearly doubled since 2009. That's a big improvement over a decade ago. But our connectivity to other IT systems is still poor, meaning that electronic files stay inside one clinic or institution rather than following patients into whatever part of the health care system they roam.

And so far, few Canadian primary care practices use their electronic records in a proactive way. Whether you're due for a tetanus shot or a blood pressure check, chances are we're leaving it up to you to figure that out. The occasional reminders people do receive tend to come from centralized programs, like cancer agencies, rather than from their primary care doctor's office. We need to up our game.

I know one practice that brought in an electronic medical record (EMR) system in 2007 and used it to more reliably monitor patients with chronic disease. They developed a profile of each patient, with codes for seventeen major chronic diseases. Using those codes, the doctors were able to develop reminder prompts for patients who had diabetes or osteoporosis, for those with serious mental illness, or for those who were due for smoking cessation talks or cancer screening. They were even able to build patient education tools into the EMR and use them to guide conversation in the office, later emailing them to the patients at home.

Examples like these don't just happen because you plug a computer into the wall. Technology makes population-based primary care much easier to deliver, but it isn't always the critical element.

Hospitals and clinics that had good workflow in the old paper systems tend to continue to do well on EMRs, and the reverse is also true. As my colleague Dr. Darren Larsen likes to say, "When you add a computer to a mess, you just end up with a computerized mess." Electronic records should offer a much more efficient way of helping organizations provide population-based primary care. But some providers may just be dumping information into the computer the way they used to dump it into the paper chart—in ways that aren't useful for pulling reports, sharing information across the system, or improving care.

Eventually, the hope is that I'll be a resource for those in my community who don't even have a chart in my practice. The population I serve becomes more than just the people on my patient list, but in the broader community as well. In this universe, anyone who's moved into my neighbourhood and needs a family doctor could be connected with me automatically. Other countries have figured out how to do this. An acquaintance of mine moved to Denmark a few years ago. As she tells the story, when she arrived she was given a number to call to set up her family's health care access. She called the number, gave them her address, and they gave her the information about her new family doctor. That was it. In population-based primary care, looking for a family doctor shouldn't feel like playing the lottery.

As a community-based service, primary care needs to incorporate elements of design that resemble those of our public schools. For example, your local practice shouldn't have a choice about whether or not its doors are open to you—which means that our Ministries of Health and regional health authorities have to work with groups of physicians in each neighbourhood to ensure that this goal can be met without causing physician burnout.

Looking beyond the people in my practice to serve my community also means developing more of a focus on disease prevention and health promotion. I might partner with the public health unit to improve the health of kids in my neighbourhood through a running program or a nutrition program, or provide outreach services to a local high-rise building where many home-bound seniors live. Population-based primary care looks at the totality of the population a doctor or team is responsible for, identifies the risks to the health of that population, and then delivers services at the group and individual level to reduce those risks. It's a daily challenge to shift our gaze outside the office to the community in which our office is located.

———

A relationship is a two-way street. What do I have a right to expect as Abida's family doctor? When I need specialist advice to take care of her, I should be able to get it—in a timely way and without having to call on informal networks. And I should be able to expect some things from Abida, too. For the system to do what she needs when she needs it, Abida needs to help me be her air traffic controller. This means that she needs to see me, or someone in my practice, on a consistent and predictable basis. It also means insisting that information be communicated back to me when she's been seen elsewhere.

That doesn't just apply to Abida. It applies to all of us. You may need to trade in some of your "choice" in some circumstances—much of which is choice you probably didn't want anyway, like the "choice" to be seen by someone who doesn't know you or can't access your chart—in order to participate in building a relationship with your personal provider and team so that they can support you when you need it.

When I began seeing Abida regularly, we had a conversation about her responsibilities and obligations as well as mine. I asked her not to use walk-in clinics, and to stop going to the emergency department unless she truly believed she had an emergency. I asked her to book appointments with me as much as possible, but I encouraged her to see a colleague on my team if I wasn't around, and I put a note on her electronic chart asking team members to send me a message if they'd seen her so that I could follow up. Abida has never expressed concern about these requests. In some ways I think she was relieved to know what she could expect from me and what I expect of her.

But there are expectations I have—of myself and of the system—that aren't yet consistently met. When Abida is admitted to hospital, I still hear about it more quickly from her than from the hospital. And I don't know how many more Abidas are out there in my neighbourhood, in need of care I should be giving them.

Imagine a system in which all family doctors consistently know when their patients are admitted and discharged from hospital and what happened while they were there, so that we could better care for them when they go home. A system where patients with multiple chronic conditions receive more intensive support from home care and check-in phone calls or visits from their primary care provider. A system where family doctors can help connect people with social services, not just medical ones, to get to the bottom of what's really making them sick—like a lack of decent housing or healthy food. A system where family doctors think about their communities, not just their practices, when they think about their work. That's what I mean when I talk about relationship-based care. It's a goal worth reaching for.

Rewarding What Matters

You have probably heard the critique that you can't improve what you don't measure. In primary health care, part of our challenge is figuring out how to measure what matters, not just the things that are easily quantifiable.

A continuous relationship with a primary health care provider can positively affect health outcomes and reduce health system costs. So we need to find ways to measure those relationships.

To me, the most exciting measurement work going on in Canada is an Ontario project called D2D, or Data to Decisions. It started as the brainchild of an extraordinary family doctor from Oakville who is a self-declared data junkie. He's made it his mission to drag us all into an era of enlightened measurement in primary care.

As a regular churchgoer who sings in the choir, Dr. George Southey had thought a lot about the parallels between music, spirituality, and family medicine. In his mind, all three were grounded in the importance of listening. And when he listened to his patients, the same themes emerged over and over: the importance of access, a caring experience, the competent delivery of medical services, and professional oversight of their health.

He'd read the research indicating that health care systems grounded in strong primary care do so much better than other systems at improving health and saving money. He called this the "Starfield observation," named after Barbara Starfield, the researcher who had done the most important work on the topic. Like so many people who see patients in primary care, Dr. Southey was convinced that the reason primary care is so significant is relationships. So he set out to measure them.

Now the story switches from the spiritual to the geek domain. What can be measured and how does it reflect the relationship? Because the patient–doctor relationship is so broad in scope, he had to figure out how to measure many different elements. Some important measures could be body-part related, like screening rates for colon cancer or the proportion of patients whose blood pressure is under control. Dr. Southey began measuring these by drawing from the electronic records that most family doctors now use. Other measures assess things like whether patients can get an appointment in a timely fashion or their satisfaction with their doctor's explanation of their symptoms.

These data can come from a simple survey. For example, if you were a patient in Dr. Southey's practice, each year—in the month you were born—you'd receive a brief questionnaire from him about your experience as his patient. Not every patient responds, but enough of them do that he can develop a picture of how his practice measures up. And since we care about system costs, Dr. Southey uses administrative databases to look at his patients' utilization of other health care services, like hospital services. With this, he's able to calculate roughly how much money his patients cost the health care system overall.

Dr. Southey was able to measure a lot of things about his practice, but he struggled with the question of how much a given metric might reflect the quality of the thing he really cared about: the doctor–patient relationship. So he began to ask his patients how well any single indicator, like blood pressure control or whether they could get an appointment the same day they called, reflects broader aspects of the patient–provider relationship we all care about, like access, medical competence, or feeling listened to. Patients weren't asked to choose between well-controlled blood pressure and a doctor who listened to them, but they were asked to reflect on how important each of those things was to them as a measure of a good relationship.

By asking hundreds of patients, Dr. Southey was able to learn about the relative importance of these things to his patients at that moment in time. The importance of each metric *to the patients in his practice* is what determines how much weight it's given when they're all rolled up together into a single measure of quality, on a score of 100.

Of course, as the priorities of the patients in Dr. Southey's practice change, the relative significance of different aspects of the doctor–patient relationship will also change. Perhaps as his practice ages, chronic disease management will move to the fore. If he cuts back his hours, access to him will be more of a focus. His method of combining the indicators couldn't remain static, so he periodically repeats the survey in order that he can shift the weight each of these issues carries in his quest to improve the quality of his care. By continuously monitoring his overall quality score, he learns what he needs to do better.

The D2D project builds on this work and is now starting to spread across primary care teams in Ontario. For the first time since I've been a family doctor, we have a way to measure quality of care that doesn't feel meaningless or incomplete to me. It's a measure that reflects more than body parts or lab results; it's a measure of successful relationships.

———

The idea that we're finally measuring what matters to patients and changing the way we practise primary care is cutting edge. The urgent question then becomes how to align the way we pay doctors with the things that matter most.

Since the early days of medicare, most physicians have been paid on a piecework basis: the "fee-for-service" model pays your doctor for each encounter she has or procedure she does with a patient. She would bill the government for each individual interaction with you—say, $30 to assess you for a possible pneumonia, or $5 to immunize your child. But by its nature, fee-for-service rewards the volume of interactions rather than their complexity or quality.

Across Canada, "alternative" ways of paying family doctors have become much more common over the last decade; in fact, as of 2013, only about a third of family doctors were still receiving nearly all their earnings in a fee-for-service model. By contrast, I'm paid mostly through a *capitation* model. I receive a monthly payment that corresponds to the number of patients in my practice, with some adjustments for age and sex. This means that I don't need to see you in order to get paid. In my view, that's a good thing if we take advantage of it by conducting some of our appointments over the phone and by spending the necessary time in dealing with a long list of concerns during a single visit. On the other hand, you can imagine the perverse incentive here: if I make myself scarce, I can in theory collect my monthly amount without having to see you at all. Ontario's auditor general found that some of this and other unsavoury behaviour does indeed exist in these models, though it's not the norm.

There are other ways to pay doctors. Some countries, and to a small degree Canada, have experimented with a "pay-for-performance" method in which physicians are paid bonuses based on outcomes, such as whether they can bring their patients' blood pressure under control or get them to quit smoking. It sounds appealing—pay for outcomes instead of, or in addition to, volume—but it hasn't been convincingly shown to improve care. It can also provide an incentive for doctors to focus on signing up healthy, educated patients who will follow their advice rather than taking on vulnerable patients who may be less willing or able to comply.

We could put doctors completely on salary, which may work well for physicians with many complex patients requiring long visits. Yet there's some evidence that paying doctors purely on salary—which frees us from the constraints of the clock—may eliminate the incentive to see many patients, which could jeopardize patient access and make waits for primary care longer.

In sum, there is no perfect way to pay family doctors. Every option encourages some behaviours we want to see yet also provides perverse incentives that we wish didn't exist. On balance, I believe that fee-for-service is a barrier to the kind of primary health care we need. Fee-for-service promotes high-volume medicine by reimbursing doctors for the number of things they do rather than the quality or comprehensiveness of those things. For example, in some parts of the country it still happens that doctors limit their patients to "one problem per visit," forcing patients to come back multiple times just to get their concerns addressed. Rapid visits for focused issues are rewarded in the fee-for-service structure, whereas spending forty-five minutes with a complex patient like Abida is a money loser.

What's the solution? Probably a classic Canadian compromise. A base of capitation or salary could encourage doctors to do more telephone and email visits rather than requiring that patients always come in for a physical visit. In my view, perhaps 20 percent of family doctors' incomes should be fee-for-service as a way to provide an incentive to see patients rather than just enrol them and then be unavailable. We also need some payments that reward group practices (rather than individual doctors) that score well on a relationship-based set of quality metrics— like the D2D model that Dr. George Southey pioneered and that has now been picked up in family health teams across Ontario.

As more and more doctors choose to practise in groups, those groups will need to take on accountability for their performance. And there's a window of opportunity for this, given that just as our populations are changing, so is the face of family medicine.

Thirty years ago, over 40 percent of medical degrees were earned by women; today, women make up well more than half of our medical school graduates. Women practise medicine differently from men. On average, we see fewer patients per day and spend longer with each patient. During our reproductive years, we work fewer hours (in our paying jobs) per week. In fact, the newer generation of male family physicians is also working fewer hours than their predecessors, perhaps reflecting a greater commitment by men to participate in family obligations. These factors will influence how doctors practise in Canada, and the models we need to build for family doctors to practise in.

Furthermore, new physicians have little interest in the "business" side of medicine. The traditional model of hanging a shingle, hiring a secretary, and starting a filing system—the small business entrepreneur model of family medicine—is falling out of favour. Today, new graduates want less responsibility for the day-to-day running of their practices, and more flexibility to care for their patients and accommodate the other parts of their lives: in fact, only 1 percent of new family medicine graduates from Canadian medical schools want to enter traditional solo practice.

To me, this represents an opportunity. If we're going to provide public support for family medicine in the form of clinic infrastructure or interprofessional teams, if we're going to pay our family doctors well for the work they do, and if those family doctors want to practise differently than their predecessors did, we should provide the supports needed in primary care and demand accountability for the things patients deserve. In my view, some things should not be negotiable: team coverage for evenings and weekends, reasonable availability for urgent appointments, and the use of electronic medical records. Though this will take some time, those records should be deployed, through such enlightened metrics as those found in D2D, to proactively manage the health of one's practice population.

Over time, we need to move to a system where we're measuring what matters in family medicine and paying doctors and teams to achieve those standards. That is a much higher degree of accountability for the way we practise than Canadian family doctors are accustomed to. I don't think this is a problem. I believe that most family doctors will find it entirely reasonable that our remuneration and the supports we get should depend on our provision of those aspects of relationship-based primary care we can control.

But some doctors may not want to be accountable to anyone but themselves for the hours they work or the way they choose to practise.

They may not want to be told that they can't take a vacation without arranging coverage for their patients, or that they have to cover a colleague's patients when it's her turn to go away. They may not feel it's appropriate that they be obliged to prove they use electronic records or to have a mechanism for reaching out to women in their practice when they're due for a Pap test. We'll need to decide as a profession and as a society whether we're prepared to continue to let that accountability be optional.

To decide that it isn't optional would represent a big change. I think we're ready. Without that accountability, I don't see how we can achieve the goal of relationship-based primary care for every Canadian.

————

The Big Idea here—population-wide, relationship-based primary care for Canada—is achievable. Our health care system would have many of the positive characteristics of a good public school system: greater consistency in the curriculum no matter which school you go to, an expectation that your local school will always have its doors open to you, and accountability for teaching the things that children need to learn. A population-wide primary care system wouldn't force you into the local doctor's practice, but it would ensure that there's a doctor in your neighbourhood.

When this Big Idea has taken hold, payment models will make good use of our tax dollars by ensuring your access to the provider you need rather than steering you to a doctor every time. But you'll also develop a relationship with a doctor or a nurse practitioner whom you regard as your personal care provider. It will be someone committed to developing a real human relationship with you, and we'll pay for that rather than for each little interaction with you. We'll also have well-established systems in place to get you access to specialty care or other resources in the community when you need them.

Building a health care system centred on primary care sounds like a simple idea. But as long as primary care remains mostly "outside" the health care system, provided by individual physicians or small groups unconnected in time, space, data sharing, and relationship from the rest of the system, we will struggle to achieve its potential. The most important building blocks are there already: a good supply of highly trained family physicians and other team members working in a single-payer system, and a population of citizens willing to engage with them. Now is the time to do even better by focusing on relationships.

BIG IDEA 2

AHMED: A NATION WITH A DRUG PROBLEM

Medicare's Unfinished Business

Just as no parent should have a favourite child, doctors shouldn't have favourite patients. But we all do. There are a few people in my practice who bring a smile to my face when I see their names on the day's schedule. Ahmed is one such person.

Ahmed is a taxi driver of South Asian heritage. He lives in downtown Toronto with his wife and three kids, and, despite a university education, he works long shifts behind the wheel. I got to know him better when I took care of his wife through her pregnancies. Her English has improved dramatically over the years, but in the beginning he would often translate for her. He is unfailingly polite. He has a lovely smile. He is remarkably articulate, not only about his physical ailments but also about his emotional frame of mind, something I confess I am not accustomed to in men of his age. I once hailed a cab downtown and he was behind the wheel. He absolutely refused to take my money.

Like so many taxi drivers, Ahmed's sedentary job has predisposed him to his current medical problems: diabetes, high cholesterol, and high blood pressure. His genetic background is another important risk factor, as people of South Asian descent have high rates of these same diseases. And although he and his wife are careful in their spending, he simply cannot support his family and pay for his prescription medicines.

Sometimes I don't see him for long periods, and when that happens I know it's because he isn't taking his medicine and doesn't want to disappoint me. I worry, as he does, about the complications he may experience in the coming decades. Some of those complications could be devastating, such as heart attacks, strokes, and blindness—and his risk is much higher because he can't afford his needed medicine.

Ahmed's situation, and stories like his across Canada, clearly illustrate the need to expand our public insurance plans to include coverage of medically necessary prescription medicine. We are truly international laggards: Canada is the only developed country with universal health coverage that does not include prescription drugs.

Implementing a national pharmacare program is the right thing to do for the health of our population, and it would actually save us money. *Lots* of money. That's why it's a Big Idea worth getting behind.

———

Like medicare, pharmacare is a simple but powerful idea. Every Canadian would be covered by a public insurance plan for medically necessary prescription medications, just as we're covered for medically necessary doctor and hospital care. The insurance could be at the national level, or at the provincial level with coordination and standards across the country.

In order to work, pharmacare must cover the same list of medications for every Canadian. A list of drugs covered, called a national formulary, is a base requirement. That list must be developed and maintained through a process that is free from political interference and from industry influence. Not every drug should be free—as in all areas of health care, we should make decisions about what to pay for based on the best available medical evidence. A national formulary would guide doctors in prescribing and patients in the choices they make about what medicines to take.

Under a pharmacare system, when you go to the pharmacy to fill a prescription, you would present your health card and receive your medicine. A single agency would purchase the drugs for our whole country in bulk, and would negotiate the best possible prices for our drugs with the pharmaceutical companies that produce them.

Pharmacare should also be designed to reduce the overmedication and inappropriate prescribing that too often take place in Canada.

It sounds good, doesn't it? So why haven't we had this from the beginning?

———

The omission of prescription medications from medicare is mostly an accident of history. When medicare was developed in the 1950s and 1960s, physicians provided the bulk of health care and hospitals were the typical care setting. As a result, today when a person like Ahmed is admitted to hospital, his medicines are covered as part of the medically necessary treatment he receives there. And yet our systems are now rapidly transforming to meet the needs of an aging population that is living longer with chronic disease, and doing so not in hospitals, but in the community. Nearly one–third of Canadian adults live with at least one chronic condition, and one of the mainstays of treating many chronic diseases is prescription drug therapy. But when Ahmed sets foot on the sidewalk outside the hospital with a prescription in hand, he's on his own.

This matters for his long-term health. Prescription medicines, when prescribed to the right people in the right dose, save lives. Insulin for diabetes, HIV medications for people who are HIV positive, anti-seizure medications for people with epilepsy, inhalers for people with asthma, cardiac medicines for people who've had a heart attack—advances like these in prescription medications have marked major improvements in the management of disease.

Beyond improving health, appropriately prescribed medications do something else. By helping people manage their illnesses effectively at home, they can prevent emergency department visits for exacerbations and complications of illness. These are far more expensive than the cost of a prescription.

Those complications represent a real risk to Ahmed and his family. Low-income people with diabetes are more likely to experience a stroke or heart attack and have a higher risk of death than diabetics with higher incomes. This gap in outcomes is even wider for patients who have to pay for their drugs out of pocket: as study after study has shown, the more people have to spend on their prescriptions, the more likely they are to fail to purchase (and therefore take) their medication; fees as low as a few dollars per prescription can deter low-income patients from filling them. The day Ahmed turns sixty-five, his risk of complications from diabetes will decrease—because seniors in Ontario are covered by the provincial public drug plan.

I know that Ahmed doesn't want to go on and off his medicines depending on his cash flow. He's forced by tough circumstances to forgo them. Of course, the human cost to him—and the financial cost to our health care system—will be so much greater if we can't help him get the medications to keep his blood sugar and blood pressure under control.

———

We have allowed a completely dysfunctional system of drug coverage to evolve in Canada. It's a dizzying patchwork of private and public payers working at odds with each other, and not in the public interest.

Many Canadians are covered by private insurance plans, often through their employers or the employers of their parents or spouses. If Ahmed had drug coverage through his employer, he would expect to pay something at the counter—often 10 or 20 percent of the cost of the prescription—but by and large, whatever I'd written on that prescription would be covered. This is because the majority of private plans make no attempt to base their coverage on medical evidence until an individual's drug spending gets into the many thousands of dollars annually. If I prescribe a drug, the plan will nearly always cover it.

As good as that might sound, it isn't. Such plans give licence to doctors to prescribe more expensive medicines when less expensive ones are just as good, resulting in high costs for no reason. Eventually, the plans will pass those high costs on to you, directly or indirectly. They also encourage "off-label" prescribing by allowing doctors to write prescriptions for cases where the drugs are not medically proven to work. And they fail to provide any guidance to patients or prescribers about the most appropriate choice for a given condition.

Moreover, the fact that many people depend on employer-based drug plans causes problems in the job market. Just as Americans can find themselves trapped in the wrong job because they need the health insurance their employers provide, in Canada drug coverage becomes a factor in people's career and job choices. A parent whose child has diabetes or the spouse of a cancer patient can't afford to lose his or her employer-based insurance. This traps people in jobs that may not be right for them, causing inefficiencies in the labour market. In the U.S., health economists have coined a term for this phenomenon: it's called "job lock."

Physicians on both sides of the border see job lock all the time. One of my colleagues recently told me about a middle-aged man who worked as a provincial-park guide in a remote part of Canada where snakes were one of the big attractions. He'd spent years educating himself on the area's history and wildlife. The park was well known as one of the few major employers in town that was able to attract people with higher levels of education.

It was obvious that the job fulfilled a personal passion in this man. As someone who'd once visited the park recalled, "To hear him speak about going into snake pits and counting the number of each sex in a 'snake mating ball' was almost enough to convince me to overcome my mild phobia of snakes and climb in."

Then cuts started rolling through the parks system, and his job went from full time to on-call casual with no benefits. Eventually, he left to take a full-time job as a cleaner in a local school because he needed the benefits. My colleague was sad to see him leave the work he loved and was so well-suited for, just so he wouldn't lose his health benefits, including his drug coverage.

Today, only about 60 percent of Canadians are covered by private drug insurance. This means that lots of people who are working—the self-employed, people who work on contracts, people who work part time, and people who work in small businesses—do not have private coverage. Nearly three-quarters of part-time workers do not have benefits through their work. Young people and women, who are more likely than older workers and men to be in part-time work, are especially vulnerable. And given the changing nature of work in Canada, the issue now extends well beyond taxi drivers and nannies. Precarious work is on the rise; more and more young people are working on serial contracts and in more than one job; and fewer long-term jobs with a single large employer are available. As our economy shifts into an age where old models of employment become increasingly rare, old models of benefits are also disappearing.

Layered on top of these private plans is the infrastructure for public plans: every province, and the federal government, also runs at least one public drug plan. Who is covered by these plans varies widely across the country. In Ontario, for example, all seniors over sixty-five have public drug coverage through the Ontario Drug Benefit Plan, whereas British Columbian seniors are covered only if their drug costs exceed a given percentage of their income.

In most Canadian provinces, people on social assistance have public drug coverage. But most Canadians with jobs are excluded from these public plans—despite the fact that they may not receive coverage through their employer—unless their costs become "catastrophic."

Catastrophic safety net plans provided by the provinces are supposed to catch the growing group of people who fall through the cracks, but these vary enormously among provinces and can be hard to apply for. The proportion of household income that needs to be spent on medicines before catastrophic coverage kicks in varies from 3 percent to 15 percent. This patchwork has meant profound regional inequality: a patient with congestive heart failure might have to pay anywhere between $74 and $1332 out of pocket for her prescriptions, depending on her age and which province she calls home.

As a resident of Ontario, Ahmed would probably qualify for catastrophic drug coverage—the Trillium program—which comes into effect once he spends 4 percent of his income on medicines every quarter. For example, on an annual income of $20,000 he would need to spend $800 out of pocket on medicine ($200 per quarter) before his coverage would kick in. That requires an upfront cash outlay that he simply can't afford. And the bureaucratic process of applying for Trillium is a barrier for him, as it is for many people—assuming they even know the program exists. For people like Ahmed who can't afford those deductibles and whose drug costs are in the hundreds rather than the tens of thousands of dollars, having only catastrophic coverage is the same as having no coverage at all.

More and more people will be in Ahmed's position in the years to come. And it isn't just the working poor. In my practice, I see plenty of self-employed consultants and other medium- to high-income earners who don't have drug coverage. When faced with moderate costs, even higher income earners have declined the trip to the pharmacy. With one in five Canadian households spending $500 or more out of pocket on pharmaceuticals in 2014, the problem crosses income lines.

Furthermore, Canadian seniors and retirees are increasingly seeing their employer-based benefits clawed back. Nearly two-thirds of Canadians over the age of sixty-five take five or more medications. The needs of Canada's aging population cannot possibly be met without appropriate access to prescription medications in the community, but just at the moment we need it most, drug coverage is disappearing.

Today in Canada, fully 22 percent of our prescription drug costs are funded out of pocket by patients, and these numbers are increasing, especially for lower income families. With out-of-pocket spending that high, it's not surprising that one in ten Canadians does not fill a prescription or take medication as prescribed because he or she can't afford to. Only 3 percent of the Dutch and 2 percent of the British have found themselves in that situation in the last twelve months. This is because other countries have universal health insurance that includes prescription medicines in their health plans. It's that simple.

As more and more extremely expensive drugs come onto the market, the number of people who fall through the cracks of this patchwork system will only increase. People like my patient Julie have shown me what that looks like.

When I realized that Julie probably had multiple sclerosis, she didn't know it yet. She'd come in to see us in the family practice clinic because she had suddenly lost her vision in one eye. What followed for her was a series of specialist appointments and MRI scans, difficult moments breaking the news to her family and friends, and the slow process of coming to terms with her life as a young mother with two small children and a chronic and potentially debilitating disease.

That should have been enough for her to deal with. But when the price tag for the medications she needed came in, she realized that there was a whole other dimension to her problem. The annual cost for the medicine Julie needs is $25,000. She's one of the lucky Canadians with insurance coverage, but like many private insurance plans, her insurance covers only 80 percent of the cost of her drugs. This left her and her husband wondering where they were going to find the other $5000 every year.

Believe it or not, Julie is one of the lucky ones, because she did find a way to pay for her MS medication. An employee in the hospital's MS clinic *whose job it is to figure out how to get medicine for patients with MS* helped her apply for the pharmaceutical company's "compassionate access" program, which covers most of the rest of the cost. (It's nice that these programs are available, but let's remember that they wouldn't be needed if the prices were more reasonable to begin with.)

There are literally millions of people across Canada who face situations similar to Ahmed's and Julie's. They are waiting to see whether they'll be able to fill their prescriptions before visiting their family doctor to discuss a chronic medical condition; they are battling with insurance companies about the copayment on their expensive medication; they are debating whether controlling their blood pressure is really more important than sending their kid to soccer camp this summer.

————

When I realized why Ahmed wasn't getting his blood sugar under control, I felt embarrassed. I was embarrassed that I hadn't figured it out sooner, and even more embarrassed that there wasn't much I could do for him. Canadian doctors see the risks every day when we treat patients who struggle to afford needed prescriptions, and we mostly feel frustrated and powerless about it. So we all engage in a series of complicated workarounds to try to help the Ahmeds and Julies in our practices.

Ask physicians you know what they've done to get medicine for their patients. When I asked a few colleagues to share their stories, one immediately recalled a man in his fifties whom she'd cared for during her residency. He had uncontrolled high blood pressure that was difficult to bring down. The clinic she was working in kept samples of new and expensive medications provided by their local pharmaceutical company representative. They tried a combination of these pills, which brought his numbers down to a reasonable range. Once the samples ran out, she wrote him a prescription for the same combination of new medicines.

"When I sent him to fill the prescription, he came back furious," she wrote to me. "He had no insurance and was simply not prepared to spend all his income on medication. He flat out refused to take the pills. I argued with him that he needed to in order to prevent a stroke or heart attack. He countered by saying that he preferred to be able to pay his rent. . . ."

In the end, my colleague made arrangements for the patient to page her once a month. She would sneak down to the clinic and steal the pharmaceutical samples for him from the clinic's medicine cabinet. This continued for over a year until the clinic no longer kept samples.

"Eventually I finished my residency, moved on, and lost track of him," she remembered with regret. "I hope he didn't die early of a stroke or heart attack."

Every day in your community, a doctor is doing something she shouldn't have to do to get medicine for her patients. Sometimes that means spending time being lobbied by pharmaceutical reps in order to get a few boxes of drug samples. (In fact, as a colleague recently pointed out, the growing number of people without reliable coverage is making it more difficult to decide which patients will get the drug samples some doctors have in their office cabinets.) I could probably do this for Ahmed, but I wouldn't be doing him any favours by raiding the sample cabinet for him. The most I'd be able to provide would be a few weeks' or months' worth of medicine that he needs to take for years. And the samples given out to doctors by drug companies are never the old, generic, tried-and-true medicines that Ahmed should be taking. Instead they're almost always the latest generation: new classes of on-patent drugs that cost a lot more but are often no more effective than their predecessors. Once the samples run out, Ahmed would be stuck on a pricey regimen with no generic equivalent, and he needs to be on medication for life. Switching him to the cheaper alternative after six weeks of samples could be disruptive to the management of his illness. Drug companies know this, which is exactly why those particular medicines are handed out in this manner.

Giving out samples is one way doctors try to help patients get their meds. Another is to prescribe an alternative to the drug that's actually needed so that patients can afford to fill the prescription. The last time a low-income parent was in my office with a child who had an ear infection, I called a community pharmacist and spent ten minutes on the phone trying to figure out what the least expensive antibiotic option was for her ear, multiplying out the length of the course of therapy by the cost per dose. The treatment I prescribed worked, but what a waste of everyone's time.

It doesn't end there. As I had to do for Julie, almost every doctor has spent hours writing letters to pharmaceutical companies asking them to give our patients "compassionate access" to an expensive drug their insurance doesn't cover. (Or even a not-that-expensive drug, but one that the patient can't afford.) Sometimes this works, sometimes it doesn't.

Some doctors choose to hang on to a mostly full pill bottle brought back by a patient who had side effects from it, knowing that someone is bound to come in soon who needs the medicine and can't afford it. Sometimes doctors buy patients' medicine themselves. Pharmacists, too, sometimes do this. One colleague told me that a pharmacist gave her patient some needed medicine for free, saying "Don't worry—I'll tell my boss I dropped it on the floor and had to throw it out."

And many doctors have confronted the moment when the best advice we can give a patient is to apply for welfare. A colleague told me the heart-wrenching story of one of her patients who was working as an attendant in a gas station when he had a stroke. When he was admitted to the hospital, they discovered he had diabetes, high blood pressure, and high cholesterol. Despite some residual left-sided weakness, he managed to return to work. His medications were covered by his work insurance plan.

The following year, the gas station closed and he lost his job. He got sporadic work in restaurant kitchens and emptying garbage cans, but his left hand and leg weakness limited his abilities and he never found a permanent job. He scraped together enough money from odd jobs to pay the rent, but could afford little else.

One day the landlady called the police, who found him confused, emaciated, with most of his teeth falling out. He was rushed to the hospital. He hadn't been taking any of his meds. A CT scan of his head revealed that he'd had more strokes.

My colleague, among others, encouraged him to go onto social assistance and he got a drug card. She vividly recalled that "He ate mushy food for *two years* as he had no teeth and could not afford dentures. Eventually, we [the family practice clinic] paid for his dentures."

He is now much improved, she tells me. "We managed to get him on permanent disability (after two refusals and a lot of running around), and found him a small, subsidized apartment. His greatest joy is being able to eat solid food. He takes his meds and his conditions are well controlled."

Stories like this illustrate how access to prescription drug coverage is a big part of the "welfare wall." This is the equivalent of job lock for people on social assistance. It refers to the fact that low-income people end up staying on disability support or social assistance because they can't afford to lose their drug coverage. When they move off welfare, they often move into low-paying jobs that don't have benefits and end up worse off. This becomes a barrier to their reintegration into the workforce.

I've had to do many of these things to try to help my patients get access to medically necessary prescription drugs. My practice isn't unique or made up of particularly marginalized people. The reality is that these approaches have become so ingrained in medical practice in Canada that most of the time we don't even notice how crazy it is anymore.

The Price Is Wrong

At the same time that millions of Canadians go without coverage, we are among the highest spenders in the world on prescription medicines.

In the fall of 2015 I participated in a panel on CBC's *The National*. I spoke about how much we overpay for our drugs in Canada. I gave the example that a year's supply of Lipitor, the branded version of a cholesterol-lowering medicine called atorvastatin, goes for about $800 in Canada. A year's supply of the *exact same drug* costs approximately $15 in New Zealand. (New Zealand has since moved to a generic version of atorvastatin.)

The example was so striking that a Canadian viewer emailed me to say that she and her husband, avid watchers of the CBC nightly news, were "intrigued" by my comment and thought they must have heard me wrong, or perhaps I had misspoken. "This is quite a dollar variance," she wrote, "and we think clarification would be beneficial."

I hadn't misspoken. Among thirty comparator countries, Canadians pay 30 percent more than the average for brand-name prescription drugs, and many more times the price compared to countries where drug prices are very low, like New Zealand. Drug prices in Canada are among the highest in the developed world.

Drug spending is eating away at the rest of our health care budgets. And since so many prescriptions are either paid for out of pocket—

meaning, directly out of your wallet—or by private employer-sponsored plans that could otherwise cover other services or even go toward higher wages, it eats away at personal budgets, too. The real scandal in this country is that we can afford to cover everyone for very little more than the amount we already spend publicly on medications. There's a lot of public money in the system, but we aren't getting good value for those dollars. Currently, we pay collectively for public drug plans for some Canadians, such as many seniors, people on social assistance, and people with disabilities. We also pay through our taxes for the private drug plans that cover everyone who works for our municipal, provincial, and federal governments. In all cases, we're overpaying for the medicines we buy with this public money. We also give tax breaks on private insurance. When you add all that up, a huge amount of public money is being spent on prescription drugs.

Why do Canadians pay so much? There are several answers. We pay too much for brand-name drugs. We pay too much for generic drugs. We pay a lot of money to subsidize private insurance. And we pay for more expensive drugs when less expensive ones would do, or possibly even be more effective.

―――

Imagine you're buying a new car. When you go to negotiate with the dealer, you know and he knows that the price on the sticker is an inflated price. Like everyone else buying that car, you're going to try to negotiate something lower. Of course, the auto dealer doesn't tell you what the last customer paid for the same car. Each deal is negotiated separately, and you never know whether you got the best possible price.

Globally, the list prices of drugs are like the sticker prices of new cars. Nobody with any bargaining power pays them. So, like savvy car buyers, countries around the world negotiate rebates on the list prices. But the drug company, like the auto dealer, doesn't publish those rebates—they're confidential deals negotiated customer by customer. We'd all be better off if prices weren't inflated in the first place, whether on the dealership lot or in the global pharmaceutical marketplace.

In Canada, the limits on list prices for brand-name drugs are set by an entity called the Patented Medicine Price Review Board. The PMPRB sets the maximum price for a new drug by calculating the average list price in seven comparator countries. It so happens that four of these seven countries have the most expensive brand-name prices worldwide: the United States, Switzerland, Germany, and Sweden. This is a big part of the reason why our list prices for patented (brand-name) drugs are so high.

Public plans regularly negotiate confidential agreements with companies to get a better price than the one set by the PMPRB, just as you would for a car. This results in an incentive for pharmaceutical companies to artificially inflate the official price of drugs, since they'll have to engage in negotiations with purchasers anyway.

Private insurers don't have any incentive to engage in these confidential deals, and the employers who pay for those private plans haven't been able to bring the issue to the table. In other words, patients with private coverage don't benefit from confidential agreements and end up paying the sticker price. So do patients like Ahmed, who pay for their medicines out of pocket and can therefore least afford the higher price.

Some policy makers have argued that maintaining high patented drug prices encourages the pharmaceutical industry to invest in research and development. But there is no relationship between drug prices and R&D spending. In fact, despite our high drug prices, industry investments in R&D as a proportion of revenues have been declining in Canada over the last decades. The more we've spent on pharmaceutical products, the less investment we've seen. Compare this to the U.K., where drug prices are substantially lower than in Canada, yet investments in R&D are more than five times per capita what we see here.

R&D is a good thing for the economy and for scientific advancement, but we shouldn't pay high prices for our medicines in order to encourage the development of important new drugs. There are other approaches we could take, including federal investments in university-based basic science research and tax policies that foster scientific research in the private sector. And we could simplify the pipeline for coverage approval when good new drugs do come on the market. Pharmaceutical companies currently have to navigate a confusing set of coverage approvals across dozens of public plans in Canada, so they'd benefit from a "yes means yes" policy whereby approval for coverage on a national formulary would mean approval across the country, in every public plan.

The reality is that drug prices are driven by what purchasers are willing to pay—and in Canada, we've been willing to pay a lot. Another growing factor in pricing is the introduction of special provisions in international trade agreements like the Trans-Pacific Partnership (TPP); these can include regulations to keep drug prices high or to extend patent protection beyond what Canadian law would normally require.

———

High drug prices in Canada extend beyond patented drugs to include generic, or off-patent, medicines as well. Canadian prices for generic drugs—those older, tried-and-true medicines that patients like Ahmed need to manage their blood pressure and diabetes—are nearly double the median prices found in peer OECD countries. Even when a Canadian generic company is supplying the product, foreign countries are getting it at a substantially lower price than we are. For example, New Zealand purchases amlodipine (a blood pressure medicine) and the United States purchases venlafaxine (an antidepressant medicine) from a Canadian generic firm at substantially lower prices than Canadians pay. And the differences aren't small: amlodipine is 86 percent lower in New Zealand and venlafaxine is up to 94 percent lower in the United States.

Generic drug prices in Canada are currently set as a percentage of patented drug prices in our public plans—and it's now the norm for governments to pay 18 percent of the brand-name price for a generic equivalent. That may sound like a low price, but it's much higher than in other countries, especially where they use tendering to procure each drug from the manufacturer that can offer the most competitive price.

The ways in which high drug prices have become solidified in our system are complex. For instance, many Canadians don't realize how the relationship between pharmacies and drug companies affects generic drug prices. When you fill a prescription at the pharmacy for a generic drug, your doctor doesn't specify which version of that drug should be dispensed to you. All companies that produce the generic pill produce essentially the same version, so for you (and for your doctor), it makes no difference which version you get. But companies convince pharmacies to stock their version of the pill—by offering to share some of their profits. In the industry, these are called "volume discounts."

If profits were reduced on generic drugs because we started to pay prices that are more in line with the rest of the world, generic companies might not continue to provide such generous support to pharmacies. So far, price reductions haven't put pharmacies out of business: the number of pharmacies in Canada continues to go up every year. But under a pharmacare program, Canadian pharmacies would probably have to come to terms with smaller price rebates—which is likely to result in a tough political fight. And unfortunately, pharmacists who own their own pharmacies or have shares in the pharmacy chain they work for are in a conflict of interest on the issue. We can only hope that these highly trained health professionals who see patients turn away from the counter when they hear the cost of the prescription will be able to put the interests of those patients first.

———

High drug prices benefit the companies that produce the medicines and the pharmacies where they're dispensed. Private insurers also do well in the mix. And to make matters worse, the cornucopia of private drug plans in Canada has resulted in high administrative overhead costs that patients and workers have to underwrite.

Private insurance is expensive: private insurance companies pay $383 million more per year for generic medications than public plans do. It's also inefficient. In 2011, Canadians paid $6.8 billion more in premiums than they received in actual benefits from private drug plans. This discrepancy stems in part from administrative costs, which for drug insurance are 8 percent in the private sector compared to only 2 percent in the public sector.

Maybe such high costs could be justified if these private plans were more effective—or even as effective—as public plans at keeping drug prices reasonable and supporting quality prescribing. But they aren't. Instead, private plans mostly just process claims and pass the cost on to you, the consumer.

As a result, private insurance plans are becoming increasingly unaffordable for employers and employees. For an extreme example of how paying for health benefits affects the corporate bottom line, we need only look south of the border. In 2009, General Motors CEO Richard Wagoner testified before the U.S. Congress that covering health costs put his company at a disadvantage in the global marketplace compared to competitors based in countries with universal public coverage. "If you keep paying more and more for health care," he explained, "it robs our ability to invest in future products and future technology, which impacts our ability to employ people." Warren Buffett has looked at the numbers too and derided GM as "a health and benefits company with an auto company attached." In recent years GM and Ford paid $1500 per vehicle in health costs for employees, whereas BMW paid only $450 in Germany and Honda paid only $150 in Japan. Germany and Japan, of course, have public health care plans to cover those workers.

The problem that American corporations experience in trying to provide general health care benefits to their employees is mirrored in Canada for drug benefits. As drugs become more expensive and the risk of insuring people for them increases, employer-based drug plans are dragging our employers down, limiting their ability to increase other benefits, wages, or reinvest in their businesses.

Of course, if we were to move drug coverage into medicare, private insurance companies would lose a chunk of business. It's no wonder that the insurance industry's association has called for a "better way" to reform pharmaceutical policy by having the public and private sectors "work together." That better way might be better for insurance companies, but I don't think it would be better for patients. A version of pharmacare that leaves private plans untouched will make it difficult—if not impossible—to achieve the cost savings and quality improvement Canadians deserve. We've seen exactly this in Quebec, where the government tried to attain universal drug coverage by leaving employer-based insurance plans intact and then filling in the gaps. The result has been staggeringly expensive. A public plan that can't negotiate lower prices because it has to share the market with private plans can't bring down the price of drugs. Instead of cost containment, the Quebec approach has resulted in cost-shifting: patients are having to pay more of their drug costs themselves and there is less bargaining capacity overall.

When you scratch the surface, even private insurance companies are struggling to deal with high-cost drugs. As a colleague who works in the private insurance industry explained to me, insurers are worried that as more new and expensive drugs hit the market, employer plans will either go belly-up or start capping employee coverage, effectively passing on the costs of medicines directly to families or to public plans. This is already happening: we're seeing an increase in the number of plans adding annual or lifetime maximums. So just when you need that coverage most, you may discover that it's run out.

The expense of private drug plans is even more out of reach for small businesses, which are an important part of our economy and often can't afford drug coverage for their employees. It's a tough expense to take on, especially if an employee needs expensive drugs for a rare condition. Drug costs are rising every year for employers, and they're likely to continue to rise rapidly. And as the costs of private plans grow, businesses of all sizes—and their employees—will have to make difficult trade-offs.

So, under a national pharmacare program, it's Canadian businesses and industries—from the small business owner who can't afford to buy insurance for her employees, to the medium-sized business that outsources the whole affair to an external company, to the large corporation that essentially runs a small insurance company through its HR department—that will be among the biggest winners. Implementing universal public drug coverage would save our corporations and families $8.2 billion annually by taking the burden of drug costs off their balance sheets. Think of the potential investments Canadian companies could make with that money. Think of how much more competitive our industries would be if they were no longer on the hook for employee drug plans.

Furthermore, private insurance plans are subsidized by the public purse: employers who pay for private insurance for their employees get a tax break on the cost of that insurance. Ironically, the subsidy is largest for employers with the most highly paid employees.

In 1994, those federal and provincial tax subsidies to employers amounted to $2.28 billion every year; with costs increasing steadily since then, we can be certain that the annual number is higher today. Putting an end to those tax breaks would free up dollars to cover people who have no insurance or to eliminate copayments and deductibles in our public plans. And since a national pharmacare program would liberate corporations of billions of dollars of direct spending on private insurance for their employees, putting an end to the tax subsidies isn't likely to raise corporate objections.

———

Apart from overpaying for our medicines and our insurance, Canadians often pay for more expensive medicines when less expensive ones would do the job. When we hear of new drugs coming onto the market, we often assume that they represent some kind of breakthrough. In fact, many new drugs are little better than their predecessors—but they do cost a whole lot more. Up to 90 percent of new drugs provide few new benefits, and the promotion of those drugs can account for as much as 80 percent of the increase from what their predecessors cost. Often called "me too" drugs, recent examples include heartburn medications and newer versions of medicines to reduce cholesterol. And we've all seen news stories about very expensive new cancer drugs that may give people only a few more weeks to live, often with a poor quality of life—but at huge cost.

But some drugs really are breakthroughs. Take Sovaldi (sofosbuvir), for example, a relatively new treatment for hepatitis C. Hepatitis C is a chronic liver disease caused by a virus. Until Sovaldi came on the market, treatments had terrible side effects and were often ineffective. Sovaldi really works; the cure rate is up to 96 percent when taken in combination with other therapies. However, at the time of its release, the price in Canada of a twelve-week course of therapy was $55,000. That's about $650 per pill. In the U.S., the price was $1000 per pill for a total cost of $84,000 per person treated.

It's true that effective treatment of hepatitis C will bring long-term savings: think of the costs cut by no longer having people with chronic liver disease in the system. And with any new drug, at least some of the price reflects the fact that bringing new drugs to market is an expensive exercise for drug companies. In the business world, failure has a price; the drugs that make it onto shelves have to pay for the ones that didn't.

But how is the price determined? Consider that in Europe, as in Canada, Sovaldi cost $55,000 for a full course of treatment. Yet in India, where the majority of the population could never pay those kinds of prices but the market is large, the price was set at $900. This is not to say that developing countries should pay the same price as developed countries for their medicines—but it does illustrate that a primary determinant of price in the world of new drugs is "willingness" to pay.

These wild variations in pricing indicate a profound truth about the prices of new drugs. We should not assume that prices reflect any rational approximation of what it costs to develop any one given product. Pricing for medications, like pricing for any other product, reflects what the market will bear. And when there are no comparable competitor drugs, the best hope the buyer has in negotiations is to maximize purchasing power. This is why countries and other large buyers that negotiate with the makers of expensive drugs get better prices. Why should Canada not get the benefit of the kinds of price negotiations that take place in other developed countries?

The Sovaldi example raises other important questions about who should be treated with extremely expensive drugs. Sovaldi is clearly cost-effective as hepatitis C disease progresses, but it's being promoted by some as appropriate for all hepatitis C positive patients. This is despite the fact that 25 percent of people infected with the virus will spontaneously clear it themselves and therefore don't require any treatment at all. At prevailing prices, broad prescribing is a huge challenge to cost-effectiveness and affordability. At, say, $900 per course of treatment, it might be a different story—especially given that hepatitis C is a relatively common disease, so that even at a much more reasonable price, a company making hepatitis C medicine would surely still make a profit.

We could learn a lot from New Zealand. In 1993, the New Zealand government introduced the Pharmaceutical Management Agency, more commonly known as PHARMAC, in response to significant increases in medication prices. It moved away from a fragmented purchasing system, tripling its purchasing power, and implemented a tendering process. Between 2013 and 2014, tendering—the practice of competitively procuring each drug from the most competitive manufacturer—led to savings of over $50 million.

We have dozens of purchasers of drugs in Canada. Even if we didn't move to tendering but focused on more assertive price negotiations by a single purchaser for the country, we would do far better. Governments have taken some steps to start purchasing some medications together. But our public plans represent less than half the market for pharmaceuticals in Canada. As long as private plans are willing to cover more expensive options regardless of their effectiveness, it's going to be extremely difficult to negotiate the best prices possible for our prescription medications. So Ahmed will continue to face high out-of-pocket spending, and his prescriptions will still go unfilled.

Prescribing Smarter

Ahmed's story is one of poor coverage and high prices. But one irony of current prescription drug use in Canada is that while many people can't afford their medicines at all, many others suffer the effects of overprescribing and inappropriate prescribing. Too much medicine can also be very bad for our health. So while we absolutely need to remove barriers to accessing needed medicines, universal pharmacare can't be a blank prescription for the nation. We need to prescribe smarter, not just more.

Canadians are taking more prescription medicines than ever before. Some of that increase reflects real advances in the world of medicine, as in HIV and heart disease treatments, for example. But in many cases our drug-consumption increases are not actually leading to better health. So it's critical that we design our national pharmacare program not just to increase coverage and reduce cost, but also to emphasize quality and safety.

Take my patient Abida who has an array of medical problems, many of which come with prescriptions. How could pharmacare be structured to limit the possibility that I might overmedicate her, or prescribe two medicines that interact badly with each other, or prescribe expensive drugs when less expensive alternatives are just as good (or better)?

Because medicines aren't covered by medicare, no government or agency is responsible for ensuring that they're appropriately prescribed.

The result is that this critical element of patient safety is not overseen. Private plans will reimburse virtually any prescription, and drug marketing to doctors is heavy. Obviously, these factors do not support an environment of responsible prescribing. For example, off-label prescribing— in which a drug is prescribed for a purpose other than its approved or intended use—poses a significant risk to health. A recent study in Quebec found that 11 percent of drugs were prescribed off-label. Of these prescriptions, close to 80 percent were not backed by sound scientific evidence.

So we find ourselves in the bizarre situation where some Canadians can't access life-saving drugs while others are the victims of overprescribing.

A national pharmacare program couldn't fix every single thing that's wrong with Canadian drug prescribing. But if implemented correctly, it would create a strong incentive for policy makers to encourage appropriate use of medicines.

Unlike private plans, which have little financial incentive to reduce inappropriate prescribing, a public payer covering drugs for the country will want to be sure that health care providers are prescribing based on the best available evidence. Public pharmacare could facilitate evidence-based prescribing through a national formulary that would list the best choices; it could mandate the adoption of error-reducing electronic prescribing tools; and it could generate vast amounts of data to be incorporated into life-saving prescription drug monitoring.

There is no single "silver bullet" that would fix the problem of inappropriate prescribing. Most of the solutions out there have been shown to be hard to implement and to have modest effects. But taken together, and alongside a culture shift toward more thoughtful use of medical interventions, the kinds of changes we could make with pharmacare would make a big difference.

I think about a patient like Ahmed, who has three chronic medical conditions, one of which is diabetes. There are dozens of drugs to treat diabetes on the market. How can I be sure that I'm choosing the most effective, and cost-effective, options for him?

For starters, it would help me tremendously if I knew that the list of drugs covered for Ahmed would guide me to the most appropriate treatment. A national pharmacare program shouldn't cover every drug for every person all the time. Instead, an arm's-length process must be established to put in place a national formulary, a list of drugs that are both economical and effective. This list is one of the best ways to guide prescribing, because physicians will want to prescribe the medicines for which their patients are covered. Therefore the list would have to be kept absolutely up to date, with the ability to remove drugs if more effective ones become available. The process must be transparent and completely free of industry and political interference. That's a tall order, but without such independence, we can't have faith that the decisions made are in the public interest.

Other countries already do this. For example, in the U.K., the National Health Service maintains a "blacklist" of all drugs that will not be covered or insured through the public system, as well as a "grey" list of those that should be covered only for certain conditions. The NHS makes these decisions according to evidence-based recommendations from an arm's-length body. This process is not without controversy, in part because there is always immense pressure for the public system to pay for expensive drugs that may not have evidence to support them. But the process is transparent. That's more than can be said for our current system.

Not everything can be solved with a formulary. What if the first-line therapies for Ahmed don't work, or he comes in asking about newer medications that a TV commercial advised him to "ask his doctor" about? Prescribing, like so many things, is an act of habit. Most doctors develop knowledge and comfort with a small list of drugs we know well, and we prescribe them over and over. A national formulary could help us develop good habits, but sometimes we need to step outside that comfort zone. And when we do, it's critically important that our information sources be unbiased. The reality is that many doctors in Canada continue to get their information about medications from pharmaceutical company programs designed to promote that company's product. We're all busy, and if a pharma rep stops by at lunchtime with free samples, a quick fifteen-minute presentation on the newest medication, and a sandwich, it's easy to listen. Yet this type of marketing is not benign. Instead of deriding these tactics, we need to use them.

The process of *academic detailing* uses the same kinds of approaches employed by pharmaceutical companies to educate doctors about prescribing, but it provides unbiased information. In academic detailing programs, a health care professional such as a pharmacist or a physician educates doctors in order to help them prescribe based on the best available evidence. The process feels a lot like what drug reps do: short seminars at lunchtime, one-on-one brief conversations tailored to that doctor's area of interest, colourful reminder cards that are left behind with key points to remember and that can be used for patient education in the office. The difference is that academic detailing is independent of any financial association with the pharmaceutical industry. These programs are usually funded by governments, research organizations, universities, or medical associations. As a result, they can focus entirely on improving patient outcomes and ensuring value for money in the health care system, not on favouring a particular company's products.

This is not wishful thinking; other countries are implementing academic detailing and other measures to improve the appropriateness of prescribing. Under its national pharmacare program, the New Zealand government tackled the issue through several different approaches. Its first national awareness campaign—Wise Use of Antibiotics—is an annual promotion aimed at reducing inappropriate prescriptions of antibiotics for colds and flu. A mix of public education tools like posters, pamphlets, campaign prescription pads, and practice commitment posters were used to guide decisions around when these medications are actually necessary. The campaign—targeted at patients and health care providers alike—has been successful, leading to a marked decline in the use of drugs that are so often prescribed inappropriately during cold and flu season.

———

Once I make my decision about what to prescribe for Ahmed, it's important that I not make a mistake. If I reach for a pen, the risk of a safety problem is much greater. I might prescribe the wrong dose, or something that interacts with another medicine he's taking. So one of the hopes we should all have for pharmacare is that it will support the implementation of electronic prescribing across the country. E-prescribing allows me to write and send prescriptions to Ahmed's pharmacy electronically instead of using handwritten or faxed notes or calling in prescriptions. The e-prescribing program I currently use warns me about potential allergic reactions and drug interactions that could put Ahmed at risk. E-prescribing can also decrease prescription errors that result from bad handwriting or cryptic faxes.

Finally, if Ahmed does end up on a newer medication, he would be part of the large group of people who can help us learn about the effects of that medicine over time. The data available through a national pharmacare program could allow us to follow and better understand patient experiences with medications. Data collection on this scale has the potential to provide transformative insight into the effectiveness of drugs, their side effects, factors that change prescribing habits, and many other questions. Providing feedback to doctors about how our prescribing practices compare to those of our peers has also been shown to be a modestly effective way to improve the appropriateness of prescribing over time, so that if my go-to choice for Ahmed isn't the ideal choice, I can learn to do better.

———

All the evidence points to pharmacare filling a real gap in Canadian health care, yet despite decades of recommendations by Royal Commissions and calls from provincial politicians, we seem to be stuck. Why?

Part of the issue has been that although pharmacare would clearly save money for society as a whole, it would shift the burden of paying for medicines from the private sector to the public sector—from out-of-pocket spending and insurance premiums to taxes. The incremental cost to public plans isn't as big as some politicians worry it would be, but it's not zero.

How much would pharmacare cost? A research study I was involved in, led by Professor Steve Morgan at the University of British Columbia and published in 2015, quantified the costs. We found that the annual savings to employers, unions, and private citizens would be $8.2 billion. Governments wouldn't have to invest anywhere near this amount, because they can get much lower prices than we currently do. Depending on whether we achieved prices similar to the best- or to the worst-performing countries, the additional cost to governments would likely be on the order of $1 billion per year. This estimate doesn't take into account any of the savings we should expect to see in the health care system as a result of people taking their medicines as prescribed. It doesn't assume cancellation of the tax subsidy for private insurance. And it doesn't assume any improvement in the overprescribing and inappropriate pre-scribing that currently take place. (Taking any of these factors into account would make the program even more affordable.) It is solely an estimate of how much more our public payers would need to spend in order to cover everyone if we got better prices for our drugs. Divide those costs among thirteen provinces and territories plus the federal govern-ment, and pharmacare starts to feel affordable.

In recent years, many governments have focused on downsizing their role and balancing the budget. So the social objective of equitable access to medicine and the political objective have appeared to diverge. Given the federal–provincial division of powers, it's also been easy for the provinces and the federal government to point fingers at each other in discussions about whose job it should be to solve the drug problem in our country. Public support for national pharmacare is high, but despite the strong eco-nomic and moral case, this Big Idea will require political courage.

Apart from the price tag, governments are pressured by organized interests. The pharmaceutical industry, private insurance companies, and small and large pharmacies would all likely see their profit margins shrink. These economic powerhouses exert tremendous political influence. Yet the alternative—maintaining the status quo—is harming the health of millions of Canadians and hampering our economic prosperity.

The savings from universal public pharmacare don't materialize out of nowhere. As the renowned Canadian economist Bob Evans has observed, every dollar of health care spending is a dollar of somebody's income. With any major policy change there are winners and losers. The winners under pharmacare would be Canadian patients, especially those who are currently uninsured or under-insured, and Canadian businesses. The losses would be reduced profits for pharmaceutical companies, private insurance companies, and pharmacies.

These groups are all entitled to advocate for their interests. But we need to decide as a nation if we're comfortable underwriting their profits at the expense of the health of our population and the sustainability of our health care system. Every other industrialized country in the world has managed to structure systems that strike a better balance than ours.

Major change in Canadian health care is rare, but it isn't impossible. If people want politicians to do something, they have to demand it. No amount of economic analysis, policy doomsday predictions, or international shaming will cut it. Until the phones of the nation's constituency offices start to ring off the hook, change will come slowly, if it comes at all. I wish that more people had time to devote to advocacy for their own legitimate interests. But as more Canadians begin to realize that they're being ripped off by unnecessarily high prices, as more middle-class people face outrageous costs and bureaucracy to have their medication needs met, and as more doctors get fed up spending their time working around a system that is fundamentally broken, something will shift. Provincial and federal ministers of health are in active discussions about this issue at the time of writing; I hope their efforts will not stop short of the goal.

It doesn't happen very often in the world of public policy that the right thing to do is also the less expensive thing to do. The economic and health case for pharmacare is clear. If access to care in Canada is to be based on need, not ability to pay, there is no justifiable reason to continue excluding prescription medications from our public plans.

BIG IDEA 3

SAM: DON'T JUST DO SOMETHING, STAND THERE

The Compulsion to Cure

Sam was a healthy man in his sixties who came under the care of a cardiologist colleague. He didn't smoke, didn't drink, and wasn't taking any medications. In fact, he was a world-ranked athlete for his age group in a competitive sport. As part of his compensation package at a powerful firm in downtown Toronto, he went every year for an executive physical. Executive physicals are often offered to business leaders as perks—they visit fancy private clinics with carafes of cucumber water in the waiting room and undergo a whole series of tests that wouldn't normally be offered in the public system because there is no evidence to support their use. Many of the tests and the doctors' services are billed to the public system, but employers pay high fees for the components of the service not covered by the public plan.

One year, despite the fact that Sam felt perfectly well, he was subjected to an exercise stress test, "just in case"—it was offered as part of the executive package of services. Some incidental potential abnormalities were identified. He ended up with an angiogram—an invasive test where dye is injected into the patient's blood vessels to look for blockage of the arteries that supply the heart. Happily, the angiogram confirmed that Sam did not have coronary artery disease. But not before he suffered a stroke on the table, a known complication of the procedure that occurs once in every one to two thousand cases. This healthy athlete will never play his sport again because he's paralyzed on one side of his body *as a direct result of a completely unnecessary test.*

You may be thinking "But what if they'd found something?" and wondering whether the risks of screening tests aren't still worth it to pick up that one cancer or undiagnosed heart condition. Our culture is so shaped by the assumption that all knowledge is helpful that people— both patients and health care providers—find it hard to accept that it can cause more harm than good. We need to stop thinking only about the potential benefits of medical tests and interventions and start talking about their potential harms.

Expensive technology, early diagnosis, and aggressive treatment can save lives—but only when properly applied. When misapplied, they cause suffering and death, not to mention unnecessarily high health care costs. It's time for us to learn the difference between medicine that helps and medicine that harms. That's why the third Big Idea is the reduction of unnecessary tests and treatments in Canadian health care.

———

Most doctors go into medicine because we want to cure illness. That means we like to do stuff that makes people get better, preferably right away. When I train residents and medical students, I sometimes see their eyes glaze over when I start to talk about things like "watchful waiting"—the art of standing back to see what the body will do about a symptom if given a little time. Or I try to describe the "healing inter-action," which is the use of a brief encounter, conversation, and educa-tion to help someone through the experience of their ailment rather than ordering tests or prescribing medicines . . . and I wonder if they think I'm a flake. Medical trainees are high performers, and they're usually action-oriented. They don't enjoy uncertainty (who does?), so it's natural for them to want a clear diagnosis and treatment plan. Low-tech, relationship-based approaches don't always feel like active options, even though they are. This often means that by the end of an encounter with a patient, many trainees want to order a test, perform a procedure, prescribe a medicine, or do some other action that helps them feel as though they can tie a bow around the interaction and consider the patient's concern "dealt with." In fairness, this isn't a perspective that ends on graduation—though for many doctors it does diminish over time.

Patients, too, often consider tests and interventions to be the mark of a thorough doctor, a doctor who cares and takes their symptom or condition seriously. During my fourth year of medical school I did a month-long rotation in a rural Tanzanian village that had few health care resources. I spent many afternoons in a small, dusty clinic with two rooms and a dirt floor, learning the ropes of tropical medicine from a pair of talented and committed health workers who had little formal education but enormous knowledge of the diseases affecting their community. The first piece of advice they gave me was this: if I wanted patients to feel that I'd helped them, I needed to give them an injection. This was what good doctors did—injections were seen as strong medicine, medicine that would heal.

Lest you find that quaint, let me assure you that in North America our thinking is no different. Good doctors put needles into skin and probes into orifices to ferret out and eliminate the problem. The more high-tech the investigations and the more invasive the solution, the better the medicine is seen to be. Why get an X-ray if an MRI is available? Why advise a patient to lose weight to reduce her knee pain from arthritis when you can prescribe a painkiller instead?

Yet often the very best thing we can do for our patients is to listen—and based on their history and our physical exam, to figure out the most likely diagnosis. We can offer suggestions for improvement that aren't drug related, and give things time to either heal on their own or declare themselves to be serious. This is sometimes misconstrued by both doctors and patients as "doing nothing." In fact, physician and patient *are* doing something—but that something isn't unnecessary tests and treatments.

I've learned this lesson over and over in my career, most poignantly in the birthing unit, where the harm of too much intervention is well documented. For example, we know that when fetal heart rates are continuously monitored while a woman with a low-risk pregnancy is in labour, the likelihood of ending up with a Caesarean section increases. This surgery has risks for both the woman (such as bleeding, infection, and damage to the surrounding organs) and the baby (such as higher rates of admission to the neonatal intensive care unit). What seems like "playing it safe" by closely monitoring the baby's well-being actually leads to measurable harm.

When I was a new recruit doing obstetrics at Women's College Hospital, there was a placard on the wall of the nursing station bearing a quote from one of the hospital's legendary obstetricians: "Don't just do something, stand there!" It was a wise reminder that when it comes to birth, the hardest and often the best thing is to resist the desire—the compulsion—to intervene.

What does it mean to "stand there"? One of the most important things we do in medicine is to accompany patients through their experience. This is central in primary care, but it's true in every single part of the health care system. Members of your health care team should educate you about the nature of your disease and what to expect; seek to understand the impact of your symptoms on your ability to function; listen to your concerns about the future; plan the next steps together; and then continually monitor you to see if things change, which might then indicate the need for a test or treatment. We should accompany you watchfully—without exposing you to undue risks. Sometimes that takes longer than ordering a test or prescribing a drug, but it's the only way to achieve health care's Triple Aim of improving your health and experience of care while keeping costs from rising.

One of my colleagues who practises palliative care thinks the phrase "doing nothing" is misleading. As he pointed out, many people falsely believe that going to palliative care means doing nothing, yet the nurse-to-patient ratio on a palliative care unit in his hospital is as high as it is on the internal medicine floor, if not higher. "We monitor different things," he explained. "We don't monitor blood pressure but we do monitor pain, for example. And we do lots of stuff for people, such as aggressively manage secretions and treat their pain." He's found that it's important for family members to understand this, because it alleviates the concern that loved ones won't be cared for once they've transitioned to palliative care. Like the decision not to test or treat, he told me, that transition "involves a detailed, often time-consuming conversation, and a commitment to follow the patient closely and adjust decision making over time."

I'm not trying to sell you on the magical ability of the body's self-healing process. There is ample scientific evidence that overexposure to tests, treatments, and interventions can do more harm than good; sometimes our patients would be better off without our "help." Consider, for example, the explosive finding in a 2015 study published in *The Journal of the American Medical Association*: patients admitted to teaching hospitals with high-risk cardiac conditions were *less* likely to die if they were admitted to hospital when many of the cardiologists were out of town at the annual national cardiology conference. Why? One possible explanation is because when the doctors were away, the patients were less likely to be subjected to high-risk interventions.

———

How have we ended up in a situation where we're too frequently exposing patients to harmful interventions? There isn't a single cause, nor will there be a single solution. Factors that have contributed to the rise of overtesting and overtreatment include the redefinition of disease, the leverage of corporations, the culture of medicine, the fear of litigation, the way we train our doctors, and the influence of patient expectations—to name a few.

When I was in training, in order to be considered diabetic a person's blood sugar level had to be consistently above 7.0 after fasting for twelve hours. In the early 2000s, a new disease known as "pre-diabetes" emerged, which includes people who have fasting blood sugars above

6.0. Today, the most recent guidelines suggest that even people with sugars below 6.0 are at increased risk, effectively creating a group of pre-pre-diabetics.

Being "pre-sick" doesn't lead to disability or death; the worst outcome is to eventually become actually sick (and this doesn't happen to all pre-sick people by any stretch). Nonetheless, in recent years we've seen the lowering of diagnostic thresholds for diseases like diabetes and high blood pressure and the emergence of "pre-disease" diagnoses.

It may be good to know that you're "pre-sick" if it helps you avoid becoming actually sick. But in many cases we don't reduce that risk—we just give you a label earlier. That label inevitably leads to more tests, and, in some cases, even treatments with side effects and unclear benefits. In my practice, I find it tough to navigate the discussion with patients who are in this "at-risk" category. How can a borderline result help motivate people to make lifestyle changes without frightening them with a label that doesn't have a clear meaning?

From a population perspective, small changes to testing thresholds for diseases and conditions can have the effect of turning millions of people into patients. When the definition of what constitutes "abnormal" cholesterol levels changed in the United States in 1998, forty-two million new cases of high cholesterol suddenly came into being. That's more than the entire population of Canada.

Of course, eating well, exercising regularly, getting enough sleep, maintaining a healthy body weight, not smoking, and not drinking would prevent a huge number of diseases and many pre-sick people from getting actually sick. But those lifestyle changes are hard to make, and harder to sustain. So it begins to feel inevitable that the health care industry will push for earlier treatment with drugs instead of focusing on non-drug approaches.

More concerning is that in the case of pre-dementia, pre-diabetes, or pre-hypertension, the current benefits to patients from earlier diagnosis and treatment are often marginal. There are exceptions, of course: Pap smears to identify pre-cancer of the cervix and genetic testing for patients at high risk of developing certain types of breast and ovarian cancer are two examples. These are the exceptions that prove the rule.

Even if it doesn't improve the health of patients, treating pre-diseases can improve the bottom line of the companies that develop the treatments. A recent study looked at expert panels who were proposing changes to disease definitions that would increase the number of individuals considered to have them. The study found that none of the panels rigorously assessed the potential harms that could result from widening these definitions. And, significantly, most of the panels had a majority of members with financial ties to pharmaceutical companies.

Industry influence extends beyond disease definition. Marketing to both physicians and patients has reached new heights, and is carefully considered and aggressive. Why? Because marketing interactions and relationships exert influence on the prescription pad.

Direct advertising of prescription medicines to consumers is prohibited in Canada. But anyone who watches American television—which is most of us—has seen the ads telling people to "ask your doctor" about x, y, or z "to see if it's right for you."

Advertising to patients is effective. Consider an American campaign for migraine medicine that focused on encouraging patients to talk to their doctors about new treatments. When the results of the campaign were reviewed, it was found that if extrapolated across the entire U.S. population, the campaign would have generated around $11.5 million in new prescriptions and almost as much for refills.

It isn't just the pharmaceutical industry that's shaping the culture of overtesting and overtreatment. The fear of malpractice suits plays a role as well, with tests and treatments used as a form of self-defence. The term "CYA medicine" isn't in the medical dictionary, but I probably learned it in my first week of medical school. It refers to "covering your ass": the act of ordering a test or doing a procedure not because you think the patient needs it, but to avoid being sued if it turns out later that you made the wrong call.

Canadian doctors pride ourselves on practising less CYA medicine than our colleagues in the U.S., where the culture of litigation and the risk of huge medical malpractice suits are extreme. Nevertheless, we can all think of times when we've succumbed to the fear of being sued rather than using our best clinical judgment. And if the fear of litigation isn't in play, there's always the fear of a complaint or even just disappointing a patient. Colleagues who work in the emergency department often talk about how hard it is to send patients home without ordering such imaging as X-rays, CT scans, or ultrasounds. A person comes in with a twisted ankle. You examine them. You know it isn't broken. We even have a set of "ankle rules" to help avoid inappropriate imaging in this situation. But that person has been sitting in the waiting room for four hours because they want to be sure their ankle isn't broken. They start to look pretty irritated when you suggest that an X-ray won't add much. And if you miss something . . . So you order the X-ray.

Our approaches to training physicians can reinforce both defensive medicine and a tendency to underestimate (or simply not consider) the potential harms of our actions. Medical trainees are frequently assessed based on their ability to conduct rigorous diagnostic assessments that consider every possible diagnosis—"What are the twenty-two potential causes of this woman's low platelets?"—but not necessarily on their ability to weigh the costs involved in those assessments. (And by costs, I don't just mean the financial ones.)

The way we pay doctors can also reinforce a culture of too much medicine. We've seen that most Canadian doctors are still paid—at least in part—on a fee-for-service basis, or piecework. In most cases, we don't get paid for ordering a test or prescribing a medication, but when it's faster to do so than to engage in thoughtful conversation with a patient, the fee-for-service model has the potential to drive unnecessary tests and prescriptions. Sometimes the link is even clearer: when physicians are paid for performing a test themselves, as is often the case for some heart tests and lung tests, for example, there's a financial incentive to perform more of those tests. And of course, in procedural specialties like most forms of surgery, the doctor who recommends the treatment will also be paid to perform it.

The risk of "supply-induced demand" in medicine—whereby having a lot of doctors around who need to earn a living generates a rise in intervention rates—is hard to avoid when we consider what leads to overtesting and overtreatment.

An American study that looked at the frequency of stress tests for cardiac patients who were recovering from angioplasty illustrates this point nicely. Current guidelines do not recommend stress tests within two years for patients who've had an angioplasty unless they have symptoms. Nonetheless, many patients are subjected to these tests. If the doctors could bill fees for the tests, their patients were significantly more likely to receive them. In other words, people ended up having more tests—some of which involve radiation—when their doctors had a financial incentive to order or perform them. Of course, these are rarely conscious decisions. Physicians are nearly always trying to do what they truly believe is best for their patients. But incentives shape human behaviour just as much in medicine as they do in any other job.

And then, of course, there's the patient.

In his iconic novel *The House of God*, read by medical trainees all over the world, Samuel Shem depicts a group of new medical residents who hit the wards in a big hospital and are indoctrinated into the practice of medicine through punitive schedules, sleepless nights, and a cynical view of patient care. The book is a caricature of an extreme universe where the higher calling of medicine is sacrificed in a daily grind of exhaustion, terror, and self-preservation—and it contains just enough truth that trainees often recognize the worst parts of themselves in it. Among the "Laws" passed down from senior to junior trainees is the notion that "the delivery of medical care is to do as much nothing as possible." As the senior resident explains to them, "It ain't easy to do nothing, now that society is telling everyone that their body is fundamentally flawed and about to self-destruct. People are afraid they're on the verge of death all the time."

Patient demand is a factor in overtesting and overtreatment. Of course, tests and treatments are ordered by health care providers, not patients. When we do a decent job of communicating the evidence about their harm, most reasonable people don't want unnecessary interventions. But in the era of internet chat rooms and expectations that technology can work miracles, individuals are more likely to ask for specific tests and treatments than ever before. This is especially true if they have a symptom without a clear cause, or a nagging fear in the back of their mind.

Living with uncertainty is hard, but when we try to eliminate it, there are real costs. People like Sam, the healthy executive in my cardiology colleague's practice, have learned this the hard way. Sam's unnecessary stress test yielded a false positive result—the test suggested a problem that he didn't actually have. This led to a cascade of further investigations, culminating in an invasive procedure that yielded disaster.

Of course, not all tests and treatments are unnecessary. But overtesting and overtreatment are significant problems in Canadian health care.

———

The most fundamental precept of medicine is to avoid harming the patient. But we spend very little time in our training talking about how that principle plays out in the little decisions we make every day.

The Canadian Association of Radiologists has estimated that 30 percent of diagnostic imaging tests ordered may be inappropriate or contribute little to no useful information to the management of the patient's case. It's hard to know if this estimate is accurate, but safe to say that a large number of imaging tests done in Canada are unnecessary. The value of testing also needs to be balanced with the risks. While radiation exposure from exams like low-dose CT scans is small, the general consensus is that even low-level radiation exposure carries some risk. That risk is often worth taking when the information gleaned from the scan will make a real difference to the patient's care. But when the benefit of the test is unclear, the risks loom larger. Furthermore, eliminating inappropriate CT and MRI scans would make a huge dent in our wait times for these important tests for people who actually need them.

Achieving the right balance in testing can be tricky. An example I deal with daily is the Pap test, a simple (if uncomfortable) screening test for cervical cancer. The Pap test is one of the best available screening tests in the world of medicine. It involves taking a tiny sample of cells on the cervix to look for cervical cancer, or more often, pre-cancer cells that might eventually become cancer. When picked up early, these cells are virtually 100 percent treatable, so in essence Pap smears aren't just a form of cancer detection but also of cancer prevention.

In my office, I often see women who've gone to significant lengths to make the time to see me in order to safeguard their health. So I understand why they find it confusing—or even upsetting—when I tell them that screening guidelines have changed, and that for most women, yearly Pap tests are no longer recommended. But it does give us an opportunity to discuss why the recommendation has changed to once every three years, and why that's an improvement.

Why shouldn't we screen every year for cervical cancer? Less frequent testing is not a cost-control measure. It's about getting the maximum benefit from screening while minimizing the risk of harm.

Cervical cancer is a very slow-growing cancer. Frequent screening increases the risk of finding mild abnormalities that the body would have healed by itself over time—often, "abnormal" cells on Pap smears disappear on their own over eighteen to twenty-four months without any intervention. The risk of too-frequent Pap smears is that once these abnormal cells are identified, further testing follows. And invasive, uncomfortable procedures such as cervical biopsies (an experience that no woman would want to repeat unnecessarily) bring on lots of anxiety and other physical risks.

In addition, too-frequent testing increases the chances of a false positive result, suggesting an abnormality that doesn't actually exist. The chance of a false positive on a single Pap smear lies somewhere between

1 and 10 percent. Of course, the more Pap smears a woman has, the more that risk multiplies. If she has a Pap smear every year between the ages of eighteen and seventy-eight, assuming a 5 percent incidence of false positives, she'd have a 95 percent chance of getting a false positive report during that time.

So it's better for women to screen often enough to pick up cervical cancer when it's still 100 percent treatable, but not so often that we pick up fleeting abnormalities that would have healed on their own. It's also better to decrease the risk of a false positive result. For women at average risk between the ages of twenty-five and seventy, our current understanding of the best practice is therefore to screen not every year, but every three years. That recommendation will almost certainly continue to change, now that more and more girls are being immunized against HPV, the virus that causes cervical cancer. In the future, the Pap smear may become a very infrequent test indeed.

Despite these clear recommendations, some doctors are continuing to perform annual Pap smears on women who are at low risk for cervical cancer. Sometimes this is due to force of habit, but often it's because the doctor, or the woman, or both overestimate the benefit and underestimate the risk of the test.

The "just in case" philosophy is tough to change for all kinds of testing. Take, for example, a study that looked at Ontario patients undergoing low-risk procedures like cataract removal or screening colonoscopy. The risks of these procedures are so minuscule that the vast majority of people shouldn't have any heart, lung, or blood tests done before the procedures to ensure that they're "fit." Instead, thousands of people are having such unnecessary screening tests, which include electrocardiography (ECG), echocardiography, cardiac stress testing, and chest X-rays. Furthermore, the incidence of these tests varies widely: the researchers found a thirty-fold difference between institutions with the lowest and highest rates of ordering tests.

Overtesting isn't just limited to screening tests. Even for people who are known to be sick, tests do harm. For example, guidelines from multiple cancer societies recommend against imaging to look for the spread of breast cancer in women with early-stage disease who feel well. This unanimous recommendation is based on the fact that the likelihood of spread is low (less than 1 percent) and the chance of a false positive is high. False positive results can lead to more invasive tests, treatment delays for the cancer they actually do have, and increased anxiety.

Despite the guidelines, a recent Ontario study found that out of twenty-six thousand women with early-stage disease, twenty-two thousand (86 percent) had at least one imaging test to look for spread of their early-stage cancer. The researchers concluded that "despite recommended guidelines, most Ontario women with early-stage breast cancer underwent imaging to detect metastases. Inappropriate imaging in asymptomatic patients with early-stage disease is costly and may lead to harm."

What do patients think about this? Many of my patients have said that they'd rather not be subjected to inappropriate testing; but for others, it seems hard to imagine saying no to a test. According to a newspaper article about the study I just described, one woman diagnosed with early-stage breast cancer was subjected to a chest X-ray, bone scan, and liver ultrasound even though the guidelines are clear that such tests are inappropriate . . . and she was glad. "I would hate to be the one percent of the population who would've benefited from the test and found out two years later that it was a little bit late to start treatment," the woman was quoted as saying.

The notion that testing can do more harm than good is difficult to accept. Over the last decade, I've had three patients leave my practice because I didn't want to order particular tests that I felt weren't warranted. In each of those cases, I thought we'd had a good conversation in which we reached common ground—until they left.

Occasionally I see women in my practice who request mammograms—screening for breast cancer—in their late thirties. (Guidelines suggest that women at average risk should start screening with these tests at age fifty.) What would be the harm if I were to order a mammogram for my healthy thirty-eight-year-old patient "just to get a baseline"?

Let's imagine that I go ahead and order the test, and the results come back suggesting a shadow that now requires further investigation. There are three possibilities.

The first possibility is that the test is a *true positive*, and my patient has breast cancer. In a person her age, that's not common.

The second possibility is that it's a *false positive*, and that further testing will reveal that the shadow on the initial test wasn't cancer. But in the process of sorting that out, she's at risk of harm. This is exactly what happened to Sam, my colleague's healthy patient whose stress test showed changes that turned out to be a false alarm, causing him harm in the process.

The harms from a false positive can be physical—as what Sam experienced—or psychological. For some people, when they discover that their result was a false positive, the overwhelming feeling is relief and joy—and they carry on with life. But for others a lingering fear remains, causing more health anxiety about a wider range of issues. One study found that even three years after a false positive mammogram result, women continued to be affected psychologically.

The third possibility is that my patient has been *overdiagnosed*. This refers to the diagnosis of a "disease" that will never cause symptoms or death during a person's lifetime. With a false positive, the patient doesn't actually have the disease. In overdiagnosis, the test result is correct but irrelevant.

Overdiagnosis turns people into patients without making their lives better. Instead, it makes them worse.

One review of all the studies on screening mammograms concluded that "for every 2,000 women invited for screening throughout 10 years, one will avoid dying of breast cancer [true positive and effective intervention] and 10 healthy women, who would not have been diagnosed if there had not been screening, will be treated unnecessarily [overdiagnosis]. Furthermore, more than 200 women will experience important psychological distress including anxiety and uncertainty for years because of false positive findings." Some of these conclusions are based on studies where mammography used older technology, but the complexity of the issues cannot be resolved only with better technology.

In his book *Less Medicine, More Health*, Dr. H. Gilbert Welch explains the problem of cancer overdiagnosis like this: in the barnyard pen of cancers, the goal is not to let any of the animals escape and become more deadly. This pen contains turtles, rabbits, and birds. The turtles, or non-lethal cancers, aren't going anywhere any time soon. The rabbits are the potentially lethal cancers that can jump out at any time and may be stopped with an early intervention. The birds, on the other hand, leave the pen in a blink of an eye. Those birds essentially represent cancer that can't be successfully treated no matter how early it's diagnosed. The rabbits can still be helped. The turtles leave patients vulnerable to overdiagnosis.

One such turtle is prostate cancer in men. It's estimated that nearly 60 percent of men over the age of seventy-nine have cancer cells in their prostates. Yet prostate cancer is rarely the cause of death for these men. In fact, the likelihood that testing will turn up a "problem" that would probably never have harmed the patient is as high as 40–50 percent. This doesn't mean that some men don't get aggressive forms of prostate cancer. But a huge number of men carry a "cancer" diagnosis that will never cause them any harm, except of course for the harm caused by investigations, monitoring, and the weight of that dreaded word on them and their families. And for men who go on to have treatment for low-grade prostate cancer, the risks of urinary incontinence and impotence may well outweigh the risks of their cancer ever causing them harm.

As we learn more about overdiagnosis, there's even discussion in the medical community about how we use the word "cancer." Our tests have become so precise that abnormalities meeting the definition of cancer can be found under the microscope that would never have bothered the person until we went looking for them. Language is a powerful tool that elicits certain reactions, which in turn activate a social—or in this case medical—script. Hearing the word "cancer" understandably evokes anxiety, fear, and a desire to treat—at all costs—the threat of this disease.

Yet sometimes that cancer would never harm the person at all. They may be better off not knowing about their "disease."

The bottom line on medical testing is this: in some situations and for some people, testing can help us to correctly diagnose disease, guide treatment, and save lives. In other cases, testing won't help the individual, or worse yet, it will cause harm. The challenge is figuring out which camp a particular test falls into for a particular person. This is a matter for medical judgment, not a mechanical formula. To make that judgment, a health care provider and her patient need to be able to have a mature conversation about both risks and benefits.

Patients know this, and they know they're subjected to overtesting. One in four Canadians report that their doctor has ordered a test or treatment that they considered to be unnecessary. Nearly a third of those people just ignored their doctor's advice.

One of my close friends from university had a family doctor for many years whom she loved, but who was very quick on the requisition form and the prescription pad. My friend and her husband joked that Dr. Bresh (not her real name) would send them to a specialist or put them in an MRI machine at the drop of a hat. They referred to the experience of going to see her as "getting Breshed," meaning receiving a huge workup for any minor complaint. Every time they went to see her, they'd have to make a judgment call about which of her recommendations seemed sound and which ones were overkill.

Something needs to change.

Slow Medicine

We all know someone who carries around a little pill box marked with the days of the week and filled with a rainbow of capsules and tablets for a variety of ailments. For some people, such treatments are of significant benefit to their health. But just as we struggle with overtesting in Canada, we also have a lot of overtreatment. Nowhere is this truer than in the world of prescription medication: often both doctors and patients seem to believe that the answer to any problem is as simple as finding the right tablet, capsule, or dissolvable powder. This leads to inappropriate prescribing, a significant problem that has almost certainly touched someone you care about.

That may strike you as ironic, given all my talk about people who need prescription medicine but can't access it. But for every example of a cab driver who can't afford his blood pressure medicine, there's a counterexample of a senior who's taking too much of it.

A Canadian geriatrician shared a case with me that illustrates the problem. She was asked to see an older woman with early dementia. The patient's daughter was concerned because her mother had lost her appetite and was wasting away. My colleague took a look at her medication list: she was taking twenty-three different medication classes per day! There were duplications (two different benzodiazepine sedative-hypnotics) and medication cascades (medication for urinary incontinence that caused constipation, and medications to treat the constipation). Several of these medications also caused dry mouth, which took away her sensation of taste and made it difficult to swallow, robbing her of her desire to eat.

They began a slow process of tapering off her medications so that she was never taking more than three pills at a time. Eventually, they got her down to ten pills per day. Her appetite picked up and she no longer suffered from constipation. (She did have to pee on a regular schedule to avoid having accidents.) She was more alert and interacted more with her grandchildren. Her daughter ended up saving quite a bit of money from reduced copayments for her prescriptions.

Overmedication isn't just a problem for seniors. From antidepressants to medications for high blood pressure, Canadians have never taken as many pills as we take today. In some cases these medications truly save lives, but in others their benefits are questionable, and sometimes they actually cause harm.

Increased use of prescription medication also has implications for our families' as well as our collective finances: in 2015, Canadians were expected to spend a whopping $34.4 billion on prescription and over-the-counter medicines and personal health supplies. That's $959 for every man, woman, and child in the country, including what's spent publicly through tax dollars, what private insurance pays, and what each of us spends out of pocket. It's *triple* what was spent per person twenty years ago. Our annual growth in prescription drug costs is top among wealthy countries, above even the U.S. And this isn't just because our prices are too high (although that's also true). The sheer number of pills we take is increasing year over year. In 2009 Canadian physicians wrote 80 percent more prescriptions than we did only a decade earlier.

Some of this medicine is clearly bad for our health.

Take the example of benzodiazepines for the elderly. This class of medication, commonly used for sleep and for anxiety, is very frequently prescribed. It includes medicines like Ativan (lorazepam), Xanax (clonazepam), and Valium (diazepam). They can be effective treatments for temporary sleep problems, but they're not supposed to be prescribed for daily use beyond a few weeks, and they should almost never be prescribed to seniors because of the risk of falls and fractures, among other risks.

Having trouble sleeping or experiencing anxiety can be distressing and even dangerous, but the benefits of these drugs need to be properly weighed against their harms.

Yet when older people are admitted to the hospital, a foreign environment where they're often in pain, they're frequently prescribed these medications to help them sleep. Many of these people then continue being prescribed such medications after they've been discharged, which can lead to their becoming dependent on them. Sleeping pills also increase the risk of memory problems, confusion, falls, fractures, automobile accidents, dementia, and even death in older adults.

The harms of overtreatment go beyond medications. In Canada, people undergo surgery for inappropriate reasons more often than you might like to think. For example, in looking at a group of patients receiving cataract surgery in British Columbia, researchers found that one in five had worse visual function *after* the procedure, and one in fifteen experienced no change in their vision—no worse but no better. This wasn't because the surgeons did a bad job; in large measure it was because too many patients who were subjected to the procedure had very high levels of visual function beforehand, making it pretty hard for their vision to get any better. And in orthopaedic surgery, despite clear evidence that most people with osteoarthritis of the knee do not benefit from arthroscopy (a knee "scope"), this procedure continues to be commonly performed. From cardiac interventions to Caesarean sections to surgery for back pain, Canadians are being overtreated even as we struggle to get timely care to the people who need it.

———

If overtesting and overtreatment were a disease, we would declare an international epidemic. Our research institutes would be throwing money at scientists seeking a cure. In the United States, it's estimated that 30 percent of all medical spending is unnecessary and does not add value to care. In a 2014 survey of American physicians, more than 70 percent reported that they believe the average physician orders at least one unnecessary test or treatment per week, and nearly half said that patients request an unnecessary test or treatment at least once per week. Canadian patients and doctors are facing the same issues.

Yet somehow we all seem to feel powerless in the face of this epidemic. Doctors may feel that the rise of patient consumerism, Google diagnoses, and high technology means that our patients' desire for medical care is, and will be, insatiable. I don't think so. If we're prepared to be open about the human costs of misapplied tests and treatments, citizens and their doctors will be increasingly inclined to ask, "Before we do this, how do we know it's actually likely to help?"

There are alternative ways of thinking about medicine, approaches that thoughtfully question the appropriateness of tests and interventions. In 2002 Dr. Alberto Dolara published a call for "Slow Medicine" in an Italian cardiology journal. As one website puts it, "Slow Medicine is to health care what Slow Food is to fast food"—a movement to counteract rapid processes that reduce quality by returning to slower, more considered, often lower technology approaches to human life. The Slow Medicine movement promotes a "healthy scepticism about the medical market," and is especially critical of the use of multiple medications for older people.

> "Economic interests, as well as cultural and social pressures, encourage both an excessive use of health services and an expansion of people's expectations beyond what is realistic, what the health system is able to deliver. . . . A measured medicine involves the ability to act with moderation, gradually, and essentially, and uses the resources available appropriately and without waste. . . . Slow Medicine recognises that doing more does not mean doing better."
> Dr. Dennis McCullough

In the first decade of the twenty-first century, the Slow Medicine approach and other variations on that theme began to gain traction. Putting in place processes to reduce inappropriate tests and treatments—of the kind we could institute under a national pharmacare program—is part of the solution. But a broader culture change needs to take place as well.

To achieve that culture change, physicians and patients have come together to launch a campaign called Choosing Wisely, which began in the U.S. and which I hope will be a game changer. Choosing Wisely aims to promote conversations between clinicians and patients that will help us choose care that is truly necessary and free from harm. As part of this campaign, medical groups have created "top five" or "top ten" lists of "things physicians and patients should question." These include such things as "Don't use antibiotics for infections that are likely viral" (like colds and most sinus infections) and "Don't do imaging for uncomplicated headache unless red flags are present" (like recent head trauma or signs of a brain tumour).

In Canada, under the leadership of Dr. Wendy Levinson at the University of Toronto, the campaign launched in April 2014 and has since been picking up steam. And at the time of writing, fifteen other countries have started their own Choosing Wisely campaigns. As each country develops and tests its own version, researchers will be able to compare the different approaches being used and help identify what works to turn the tide.

In some cases, curbing overuse is bound to save money. In others, it will reduce wait times. But these aren't the driving goals of the campaign. Its focus on quality and safety is particularly important because health care workers and patients aren't likely to be moved by a campaign for system sustainability; they're rightly more motivated by patient well-being than economic incentives. This is a good thing—and yet without prudent use of health care resources, doctors won't be able to help patients.

Of course, a list is just a list. One thing we know about behaviour change is that telling people what to do—or not do—isn't enough. The real challenge is not just identifying the practices that need to be stopped or curbed, but implementing changes in our clinics and hospitals and then measuring our successes and failures to learn what works. Some places are experimenting with financial incentives whereby groups and organizations are rewarded for improving quality and value. Many others are using their information technology systems to support good stewardship: for example, one health organization in the U.S. has reported a 70 percent overall decline in unnecessary Pap tests as a result of using automated alerts in its computer system.

As part of the Choosing Wisely initiative in Alberta, physicians and universities are working to achieve the goal of never requesting imaging for lower back pain unless certain red flag symptoms are present. At North York General Hospital in Toronto, the implementation of Choosing Wisely Canada recommendations resulted in a 40 percent decrease in tests ordered in the emergency department, without any observable change in patient outcomes. The decrease in unnecessary test ordering led to annual projected savings of over a million dollars, allowing the hospital to invest in other projects. And a group of motivated and passionate Canadian medical students have launched their own list of things that medical trainees should question regarding tests and treatments.

Training in the area of reducing harm and waste should be required education for every doctor in every specialty. Surrounded by colleagues and in a safe space for reflection, we need to acknowledge, as a profession, that even good tests and drugs, when used on the wrong patients or at the wrong interval, harm people. We can't just lay the responsibility on patients who read something on the internet. We need to wrestle with the many complex reasons why, every day in our own practices, we make those little choices to tick that box or prescribe that antibiotic.

Unlike some of the other Big Ideas in this book, there is no single lever to pull to make this culture change happen. It isn't about delisting items from the public plan or demanding a full stop to various forms of tests or interventions.

The assumption of the Choosing Wisely approach is that the key mechanism for change lies in communication between health care providers and patients. While doctors often order tests and write prescriptions of their own volition, they also often do so because patients want it: when asked how they'd behave in specific situations, 36 percent of American physicians surveyed said they would accommodate patients who expressed a strong desire for a test, even if they knew it was unnecessary.

Is this "right"? Should physicians push back against patients who, after full discussion of the risks and harms, still want a test or treatment? This is an ethical conflict that recurs in every medical office. What do I say to my patient whose mother died of ovarian cancer and who wants a pelvic ultrasound? The evidence is clear that ultrasound isn't a good screening test for ovarian cancer . . . but she lies awake at night worrying.

There is no right answer. Sometimes I tell patients that I'm just not comfortable doing it. But I find that when I do a good job of explaining why, the demand decreases considerably. When a fifty-five-year-old woman with no risk factors for osteoporosis requests a bone density scan because her friends have had one, I get defensive. I pull out the guidelines and, with some fear in my heart, begin to explain why she doesn't need it until age sixty-five. I don't want her to be angry. I don't want her to think I care less about her than her friends' doctors care about them. Imagine my delight when, having looked at the little table that indicates she doesn't need one, she smiles and says "Great! One less thing to do."

There's a fine balance between giving patients enough information to make an informed choice about a test or treatment and burdening them with too much. Choosing Wisely Canada encourages people to ask their physicians four questions that can help initiate conversations about unnecessary care: *Do I really need this test, treatment, or procedure? What are the downsides? Are there simpler, safer options? What happens if I do nothing?*

A friend recently lamented that the pamphlet his doctor gave him about his options for an eye problem was outdated and hard to understand.

He searched the internet, but his screen clogged up with information from American vendors that were selling the surgery and the equipment surrounding it. "That information was not only not helpful but misleading and confusing," he wrote to me. Finally, through the U.K.'s National Health Service, he found an online tool called a "decision aid" that walked him through the process. He found it immensely helpful in preparing him to talk to his doctor about his preferences.

When there's no single top choice among screening or treatment options, a decision aid offers a formal way of helping you think through your situation. It usually begins with a series of questions that help identify your personal preferences and priorities, and then it provides you with information about your options. Whether it's a pamphlet, video, app, or online tool, a decision aid can really improve the quality of communication between doctors and patients. The Ottawa Hospital Research Institute even has a Decision Aid Library Inventory that covers issues ranging from acne to osteoarthritis.

And unsurprisingly, the use of decision aids has been shown to reduce the number of patients choosing procedures like elective surgeries—probably because they help people get a better sense not just of the potential benefits, but also the potential harms.

Beyond decision aids, there is much we can do to help citizens become more engaged in reducing harmful care. This was illustrated in the recent EMPOWER study (Eliminating Medications Through Patient Ownership of End Results). The researchers wanted to find a way to reduce the use of dangerous sleeping pills in the elderly, so they designed a "patient empowerment intervention"—an eight-page booklet containing information about the risks of medications and drug interactions as well as peer stories and recommendations for tapering down medication doses. Participants in the study were encouraged to discuss the issue with their doctors.

Sixty-two percent of the "empowered patients" discussed stopping their sleeping pills with their doctors or pharmacists at some point during the six-month follow-up period, and 27 percent of them stopped taking their sleeping pills. Compare this to a 5 percent success in stopping sleeping pills with our usual approaches.

People are increasingly trying to be informed consumers in other aspects of life. Why not in our own medical care? If every professional group in health care were to take the issue of overtesting and overtreatment to heart, if every patient association were to examine its implications, if our universities incorporated it into curricula, and if our internet forums and Twitter feeds encouraged the conversation, we might finally move into a more enlightened era of health care. We would measure the value of our work not by the number of things we do to people, but by the real improvements in their health.

The purpose of medicare, after all, is to give citizens the care they need when they need it, regardless of ability to pay—so that they can live productive lives. Care that doesn't meet that bar should be of no interest to us. Let's get rid of it.

BIG IDEA 4

SUSAN: DOING MORE WITH LESS

The Revolving Door of Health Care

Susan is a seventy-five-year-old widow who lives alone in a medium-sized community in Saskatchewan. Her kids moved to the big city for work, so she's on her own, but she has lots of friends in the neighbourhood and an active social life. As each decade has passed, she seems to have accumulated another diagnosis: diabetes in her late fifties, lung disease in her mid-sixties from smoking in her youth, a heart attack at the age of seventy-two followed by bypass surgery, and osteoporosis on her seventy-fourth birthday. Like so many of my own patients, Susan takes eight different medications, sees three different specialists, and needs to be on top of many elements of her own care. She does pretty well, and she never misses her bridge game on Tuesdays. Her neighbours help her with gardening in the summer and snow shovelling in the winter.

It's winter now, and Susan gets a cold. She feels very unwell, and is having a hard time eating and drinking. After a few days she starts to feel weak, so she decides to see her family doctor. He is away in Florida for two weeks. The message on the answering machine says that if she can't wait for his return, she should go to the local emergency department. Two days later, feeling increasingly terrible, she goes to the ED, and is admitted to hospital because she's dehydrated.

While in hospital, Susan has trouble sleeping in a strange hospital bed. She's prescribed a sleeping pill by the busy doctor on call. She becomes confused and groggy due to the pill, and when she gets up in the middle of the night to pee, she falls and breaks her hip. Two days later she has surgery to fix her hip. Post-operatively, her blood pressure is low, so the doctor stops her blood pressure medications. She leaves the hospital without a prescription for those medications, and so doesn't restart them.

A week after coming home from hospital, Susan sees her family doctor, who has no idea what happened to her in the hospital. (He'll probably receive a discharge summary by snail mail from the hospital in a few weeks' time.) But he does notice that her blood pressure is high despite the medications he was prescribing—he doesn't realize that these were stopped in the hospital. So, after ordering a bunch of heart tests that were already done last week when she was an inpatient, he refers her to a cardiologist.

The wait time for the cardiologist is three weeks. In the interim, Susan has a second heart attack and returns to the hospital. Her heart has been damaged from the heart attacks: it can't pump effectively, so her lungs fill up with fluid, causing her to have trouble breathing when she does even the most basic household tasks. This is known as congestive heart failure. When she's admitted to hospital again for her shortness of breath, her kids decide to put her on a list for long-term care because she's not able to manage at home any longer. But there are no beds available in long-term care, so she stays in a hospital ward, waiting and becoming less and less functional and more and more dependent.

After many weeks, Susan gets a spot in a long-term care home. Her heart deteriorates during the next year. Whenever she becomes very short of breath she's transferred to the hospital via ambulance. She's admitted every time and treated for a few days until her shortness of breath improves enough that she can be sent back. While in hospital she's asked a few times whether she wants "heroic measures" if her heart gives out, and she says no. But when it becomes very hard for her to breathe one night in hospital, her children ask the team to intervene. Susan is hooked up to a breathing machine. She dies in the intensive care unit following a three-week stay.

Any doctor will be nodding his head as he reads Susan's story. Even as our patients struggle with wait times in parts of our system and we worry about system sustainability, we also see enormous waste of resources, duplication, and inefficiency throughout the system. Conventional wisdom has held that wait times can be reduced with more resources: more doctors, more operating room time, more equipment. That's not what Susan needed. She needed help managing her health problems at home; she needed prompt access to primary care; she needed better communication between the hospital and her family doctor; she needed support to manage the entirely predictable exacerbations of her chronic illness without having to go to the hospital. Susan didn't need more health care—in the end she got more health care than most of us would ever want. She needed *better* health care, and she needed clear goals so that the care could be matched to those goals.

Susan's story is not uniquely Canadian. It isn't caused by the publicly funded nature of doctor and hospital care in Canada. And we are increasingly recognizing that it isn't caused by a lack of resources. In most parts of our health care system, we don't need more money, more doctors, or more fancy machines. *What we need is to better organize the resources we have.*

Money is becoming scarcer in health care. That scarcity may not necessarily be a bad thing. As Ontario's former deputy health minister Michael Decter has said, infusions of money into the Canadian health care system often haven't bought the kind of change we need. Instead, more money has tended to buy "either more of the same or actually the same with higher pay attached." Across the developed world, health care costs have been consistently rising over the last many decades. You might reasonably assume that as our health care spending increases, our health improves and we live longer. But it isn't how much you spend that matters, it's how well you spend what you have.

In countries that spend very little on health care, small investments can make a big difference in life expectancy. But beyond a certain point, spending on health care clearly doesn't lead to longer life for a population. Improvements for dollars invested are rapid until about US$2000 in spending per capita. Beyond this amount, additional gains are much more gradual and not as closely correlated with actual expenditures. This is especially clear when we see countries like Canada spending just over CAD$6000 per capita every year on health care. The U.S. spends almost twice as much by comparison (factoring in purchasing power parity) for nearly three fewer years of average life expectancy.

If we've reached the point where additional investments aren't helping us live longer or may actually be harming us, as they did in Susan's case, we need to reconsider. That's why the Big Idea in this section is to do more with less. We need to seek health care improvements that give us better value for money, by reorganizing the way we deliver care.

Of course, we don't just spend money on health care to extend life. We want better quality of life, relief of symptoms, rapid access, and many more outcomes that can't be measured in decades or even months. And when wait times are long or care seems inadequate, it's a natural reaction to think that more resources are the solution. Too long to see a doctor? Add more doctors! Too long to get a scan? Add more machines!

Those measures don't solve the problem—because the problems lie in the design of the system itself.

Let's take the movement to reduce wait times as an example. In 2004, as part of the Health Accord, the premiers and the prime minister vowed to "fix medicare for a generation," in part by addressing long wait times in five priority areas: cancer care, cardiac care, knee and hip replacements, cataract surgery, and advanced imaging (CT and MRI).

A great deal of money was invested across the country. Surgical-care wait times for many procedures improved, but the wait times for CT and MRI stayed the same—and even increased in some parts of the country. Why?

Surgery wait times were reduced when, along with the extra money invested, the care was reorganized. Interprofessional teams were introduced, new ways of managing queues were put in place, and checklists were applied to ensure that everyone waiting for a procedure was actually an appropriate candidate for it.

But in the case of CT and MRI scans, mostly what we did was buy more machines and run them longer through the day and night. In fact, in 2009, Canadians received over four million CT scans and 1.4 million MRI scans—a 58 percent and a 100 percent increase, respectively, from pre–Health Accord numbers. This brought us close to the OECD average in number of CT and MRI scans per capita—less than France, but more than Denmark or the Netherlands. Yet wait times are still a challenge in some regions, particularly for MRIs. In 2015, the Wait Time Alliance reported that less than half of the populations of P.E.I. and Alberta had access to non-urgent MRI scans in under eight weeks.

Lots of money didn't solve our wait-time problem. There was, no doubt, a big backlog of cases. But that's not the whole story. A study commissioned by the Government of Saskatchewan around the time the Health Accord was being negotiated found that at least 30 percent and up to 50 percent of imaging exams were performed for reasons not based on sound evidence. The report concluded that a very substantial proportion of the imaging being done in the province wasn't worth the cost or the increase in patient exposure to radiation.

Simply upping the number of machines doesn't guarantee a wait-time reduction. It may just increase the number of inappropriate tests being done, and it certainly won't lead to a reduction in waste. And reducing the volume doesn't necessarily mean that we'll reduce only the inappropriate tests—restricting volumes can also reduce access to much-needed services.

Unless we reorganize care and make better decisions—ensuring that only those who really would benefit from a scan are on the list and centralizing access to the available resources so that the queue is organized—*the demand will just rise to meet the supply.*

———

Local culture and variety are good if you're interested in the arts scene in a neighbourhood. But if you're having surgery, you want to know that your procedure will be performed in a way that adheres to evidence and standards, not the preferences of the team that happens to be operating that day. One of the major reasons why reorganization of care is so important is that it can help us address the issue of variation. Like many Canadian families, my family has experienced the reality of care variation first-hand.

When my father-in-law, Murray, was diagnosed with dementia, we were all sad, but none of us was surprised. His three sisters had suffered with the same disease, and we'd seen early signs for quite some time. What followed was an extremely difficult time for my mother-in-law, who kept him at home as long as she could. Eventually, it became too much for her. Murray had become aggressive, yelling at her and behaving unpredictably. He'd pace the halls in the middle of the night, interrupting her sleep. He'd become confused and paranoid, thinking she was a stranger and demanding over and over to see his wife. I still remember listening to my partner, Steven, on the phone with his dad, assuring him over and over that the woman he was with was indeed his wife of fifty years, not an imposter. Steven's mother had to grapple with the question of whether she was comfortable having her husband take antipsychotic medication to try to control his behaviour. Eventually, the difficult decision was made to move Murray into a facility, where the same question arose.

The use of antipsychotic medications for residents of long-term care is controversial, and a striking example of variation in care. For some residents, these medicines may help manage the behavioural symptoms of dementia, such as agitation and aggression. But they often have side effects including sleepiness, a risk of falls, and even an increased risk of death. It's hard for family members of people in long-term care homes to see their loved ones having a difficult time communicating or being sedated during the day. There are other ways to control aggressive behaviour, but they can be challenging to implement and require high levels of staffing, training, and commitment on the part of the leadership and staff of long-term care facilities. Sadly, drugs are easier and less expensive.

In some long-term care homes in Ontario today, the proportion of residents over age sixty-five being prescribed antipsychotic medications is zero. In others, it's more than two-thirds. Some of that variation could be due to differences in patient populations, but not all of it.

Infection control included?

My mother-in-law decided that it would be better for Murray, and his caregivers, if he took the antipsychotic medication. For him, that was the right decision. But the nature of the conversation, the way the options were presented to her, and how much power she felt she held would probably have differed in every long-term care facility across the country.

There are many other examples of care variations in Canada. For example, survival after stroke varies substantially from province to province, depending on whether the province has adopted evidence-based systems of care.

People with diabetes who live in northern or rural areas are more likely to experience such complications as kidney failure and blindness than are people who live in urban areas. Women with invasive breast cancer in Newfoundland are nearly three times more likely to have a mastectomy than women in Quebec with the same diagnosis. The likelihood that women will have a hysterectomy also varies significantly depending on where they live. The list goes on.

Of course, variations in care might be understandable in cases where we don't know what the best practice is, or where particular populations have different preferences or values regarding the care they receive. But too often, that's not the case. We know what "best practice" looks like for a wide range of cancers, heart disease, stroke, diabetes, and a host of other health issues. Yet we apply that knowledge inconsistently. This isn't usually due to an under-resourcing of the health care system. Instead it's about care that is poorly organized and delivered. Canada has been called a "nation of pilot projects" because we have difficulty moving from the trial stage to the permanent change, from the local example to the system-wide difference.

Variations in care matter. If doing things differently saves lives or money or both, we should work to reduce variation. This requires us to understand who the big users of the system are, what drives their experience of it, and where the costs reside.

———

A principle of service in any industry is to understand who your customers are. If you work for a company that makes yachts, you probably don't need to do much research into the needs of low-income people who live in land-locked regions. Health care is no different: while the system should meet the needs of every Canadian, it helps to understand the needs of the people who use the system most.

Canada looks very different today than it did in the mid-1990s; in the coming decades it will look different still. According to current projections, by 2041 nearly one-quarter of our country's population will be over sixty-five. This shift isn't the same across the country: because birth and immigration rates differ among communities, some provinces are aging faster or more dramatically than others. For example, in 2015, seniors represented 19 percent of the population of Nova Scotia but only 12 percent of the population of Alberta.

Aging alone won't bankrupt the health care system. But as people age and live longer with multiple chronic diseases, we do need to design services differently. Susan's story illustrates this need perfectly. In her case, poor communication between different parts of the health care system, an overreliance on hospital care, and the lack of a treatment plan for her chronic health conditions left her with lots of health care but not much health. Only one in four Canadian seniors with a chronic condition reports having received help with creating a general treatment plan. No wonder people end up cycling in and out of emergency departments.

A physician friend shared a story with me about his aunt, who's in her eighties and recently had a knee replacement. When he asked her about her experience, she responded that the hardest part was the unexpected pain she was experiencing as part of her recovery. "Didn't they warn you that it would hurt afterward?" he asked. "I guess so," she said, "but it didn't really hurt before the surgery."

My friend was dumbfounded. "If you didn't have any pain before your knee replacement, why did you have the surgery?" he asked.

"Because they told me I needed to," she responded.

On further questioning, my friend learned that his aunt had seen her family doctor about the knee discomfort she felt when she walked around or got down on the floor to pray. The family doctor had advised her to take Tylenol, which worked quite well; it allowed her to carry out her daily activities and do all the things she wanted to do (in some cases with a few modifications, such as sitting on a chair rather than on the floor to pray). But the family doctor had also referred her to a specialist, and when X-rays confirmed that the severe arthritis in her knees made her a candidate for a knee replacement, she was put on a wait list for surgery.

At the end of it all, she had a new knee. But it turns out that she'd been doing just fine with the old knee. She hadn't understood—and this wasn't her fault—that the point of a knee replacement is to reduce a person's pain so that they can function.

Stories like this carry a sobering message as we look toward an increasing proportion of seniors in Canada. It's wonderful that an overwhelming 97 percent of Canadian seniors say that they're satisfied or very satisfied with life. They also rate their health highly in terms of their ability to function: when it comes to their vision, hearing, speech, mobility, dexterity, feelings, cognition, and pain, most don't feel that they often have difficulties with activities. So rather than just throwing more (and more expensive) care at seniors, we need to learn to provide them with the care they need to function well and enjoy their lives.

Age is an important factor in health care use, but it's not the only factor. The health needs of people from different genetic backgrounds can vary widely, and as the source countries for immigration to Canada continue to shift, we have to pay attention to what this means for the system overall. For example, between 2002 and 2011, the highest numbers of new Canadians came from the Philippines, China, and India—and heart disease, high blood pressure, and diabetes are important risks for these populations.

This is not to say that Asian Canadian immigrants use more health care than other groups. In fact, when they arrive in Canada, first-generation immigrant adults are generally healthier than Canadian-born adults. It's just that their particular care needs may be different. If a hospital or a primary care group serves high numbers of new Canadians, providers will begin to see corresponding patterns in health care use that reflect the particular needs of those groups. We need to be able to respond to those kinds of shifts by reorganizing our resources.

Aging and the changing source countries for immigration are two factors that help us to understand the needs of health system users. Another is increased use of technology.

"Oh, the internet? Is that thing still around?" I like to joke about my technophobic side when someone else has to back up my phone for me. With virtual culture on the rise in every industry in our economy, it shouldn't surprise anyone that Dr. Google has replaced a call to someone like me as the first reaction to a colourful rash, lump in the groin, or cancer scare. Moreover, as Dr. Eric Topol, author of the terrific book *The Patient Will See You Now*, has observed, "Instead of just looking up symptoms, as has been the case with the Internet [for] over 20 years, we're about to move into an era when people will also have objective data (through sensors, labs, imaging, genome sequence) that will empower them to be highly active participants in their diagnosis and care."

Patients want to be treated not as passive recipients of care, but as true partners whose time and input is just as valuable as their doctors'. They want convenience: care close to home, available 24/7 and by email or telephone. They want to be seen in a reasonable time frame, and barring exceptional circumstances, they want to be seen at the time of their appointment. They want to be "e-patients," a term coined by a patient advocate who calls himself e-Patient Dave: empowered, engaged, equipped, and enabled. Dave began blogging about his experiences in the American health care system when he was in treatment for metastatic kidney cancer. He's since become a full-time activist, advocating for greater involvement of patients in their own care and for personal health-data rights. His book *Let Patients Help!* is a manifesto for participatory medicine.

The importance of health literacy—people setting and participating in achieving the goals of their own care—cannot be overstated. What is the value of giving people treatment plans if they don't know how to use them or the plans don't work in the context of their lives? The digital revolution has helped people learn about their health and has the potential to help them make decisions more effectively with their doctors.

E-Patient Dave predicts that it will take only about a generation to completely arrive at a new reality in the e-patient movement. From genetic tests that help us understand how our DNA influences our health risks to the uptake of wearable devices that measure the number of steps we take each day, technology continually brings new opportunities to understand and interpret our health. Still, how much this "quantified self" will actually improve health outcomes is unclear to me. In some areas it may give us more data than we have the wisdom to deal with—and if we're not thoughtful about its application, it could lead to unnecessary treatments, not to mention privacy risks. But people are turning to these technologies as a way of increasing their engagement with their health, and that's an interest that should be respected. In the information age, appropriate use of less expensive and more empowering self-care of all kinds will take its rightful place in the spectrum of health care.

Not every aspect of improving the patient experience needs to revolve around fancy technology. Health care remains a human industry, where the little things make a big difference to people's experience. Cleanliness of waiting areas. Being looked in the eye. Having people explain what they're doing and answer questions. Being given enough time with a health provider. As we strive to reorganize care delivery, we'll see increasing standardization of the processes that drive care, but care that's standardized doesn't have to be impersonal.

The imperative to do more with less is not about reducing health care staff or making their work more precarious. Too often, attempts to reorganize care have made things worse for those who are already the lowest paid and have the worst working conditions. Instead, by engaging everyone—from the staff who clean the floors and serve the food to the hospital CEO—in improving the way we organize care, we can do better for patients without putting our health care workers at risk.

Something as simple as a chair can make a big difference. One patient group, Patients Canada, found that many hospital emergency rooms had chairs for the patient and triage nurse, but no third chair for the family member or friend who often brought the patient to the hospital and knew important information that could be of use to the care team. A place for the family member would not only benefit the patient; it would also help triage nurses gain more insight into the patient as they decided on next steps. More hospitals are now placing that third chair in the triage area of their EDs. Simple, concrete things like this show a willingness to do better.

A system that serves the needs of older and more empowered patients would be terrific. It also has to be affordable. So if we want to reduce costs or hold them constant, we need to understand where our health care dollars go—and it turns out that our spending is concentrated among a small group of people who use the system heavily. In Manitoba, for example, 1 percent of the province's health care users account for 35 percent of spending on health care, including drugs, physicians, and hospitals.

This isn't just a Canadian phenomenon. It's also true in the United States and elsewhere. We call these people "high needs, high cost" users of health care, and they're the topic of much discussion at health care conferences and in government offices.

What makes someone become a "high cost" user of health care services? Imagine that you experienced a catastrophic event, like a cancer diagnosis, or a major car crash, or the birth of a preterm baby. You'd suddenly need a lot of health care.

Many of those who make up that 1 percent use the system intensively for a brief period, then either they get better and return to a lower level of spending or they die. Of the top health care users in Ontario, only 45 percent remained in that category after the first year, and only 33 percent remained after three years.

It's that 30 percent—people whose high-intensity needs are chronic—who strain the system most. Some don't have a clear diagnosis and are being extensively "worked up," undergoing lots of tests and investigations and specialist appointments. Others are living with mental health problems or addictions that make it hard for them to follow through with treatment recommendations. Still others are frail, medically complex, or have a severe, relapsing condition. When they experience exacerbations of their heart failure, or chronic lung disease, or kidney disease, they're admitted to hospital, tuned up, and then discharged home again, only to be readmitted months, weeks, or even days later. In Canada, one in every twelve hospitalized patients is readmitted within thirty days. (And in the U.S., it's one in eight.)

These are people like Susan.

Too often we see patients like Susan cycling in and out of the emergency department or the inpatient hospital simply because their underlying issues are never fully addressed and they have nowhere else to go. They spend hours, days, or weeks waiting to be seen by health care providers and have to retell their stories over and over again. They pick up infections and experience complications from the care they receive. And when they get to the end of life, we throw increasing amounts of resources at them instead of helping them die in a dignified way.

Ask any doctor you know where they want to die. I'd bet they'll answer "Not in the ICU, with tubes down my throat and a team pumping on my chest." Most of us who've witnessed the inhumanity of futile medical care—which is everyone who works in the field—want nothing to do with it for ourselves or for our loved ones. Did Susan want it? Did we ask her?

We need to focus on people like Susan—older people with multiple chronic conditions, including at the end of life. If we can improve their health, give them a better experience of care, and control the costs they generate in the system—the Triple Aim—we'll be doing more with less.

What Better Looks Like

The challenge we face is complex: an aging population that wants greater convenience, autonomy, and engagement, and better health at a lower cost. This challenge won't be met by putting more money, whether public or private, into the system. We need to develop new ways of doing things that aren't just about spending more. Here are just a few examples of what that can look like.

1. Cue the Queue

One of the biggest challenges we face in Canadian health care is wait times for elective procedures and appointments. In almost every case, we can reduce waits without spending more if we use a centralized intake process for specialty services.

When I first started my practice a decade ago, if I had a patient who needed a knee replacement, I'd refer him or her to the orthopaedic surgeon whose name I knew. That surgeon kept his wait list in the top drawer of his secretary's desk. If he went on vacation for the month of August, the wait list just grew.

Now, as a result of the concerted effort to reduce wait times in many parts of the country, when I refer a patient with late-stage osteoarthritis of the knee, that person is seen within a few weeks by a nurse and a physiotherapist. These highly trained professionals educate patients about the nature of osteoarthritis, teach them exercises to improve their pre-operative strength, counsel them on the importance of weight loss, and use a checklist to determine whether they're good surgical candidates. If they are, they can either wait for the surgeon of their choosing or see the next one available.

Let me illustrate this important point about the next available surgeon. At six p.m., when I'm rushing home to my hungry six-year-old, I sometimes stop at the grocery store. I grab whatever I need and head for the checkout line. And then I play the guessing game. Which line shall I choose? If I get it right, I'm home in twelve minutes. If I get it wrong, and I'm in the training line, or behind the teen counting coins from his pocket, it's twenty minutes. Now, if I make the same stop at the bank, I get in a single line—just one line—and am served quickly by the next available teller. The banks have figured out the beauty of applied queuing theory. Grocery stores have not.

By adopting the bank-line method and instituting a single common queue, we've reduced wait times and increased the appropriateness for surgery of those patients who are awaiting surgical consultation. And because groups like the Wait Time Alliance insisted on actually monitoring wait times, we've been able to measure our progress and identify when things start to go off track.

There is no reason why this model can't be applied to the majority of specialty care. If you have two specialists in a geographic region who offer the same services, you can do centralized intake. What's required is a willingness on the part of specialists to give up "ownership" of their wait lists and a willingness on the part of referring family doctors and patients to move away from the notion of a referral as a personal introduction. We also need to identify the kinds of specialty care where expertise can be pooled.

This concept makes some patients and doctors uncomfortable. Don't we all have the right to be treated by someone we trust? Certainly. But most patients who see a specialist do so on the recommendation of their family doctor or a friend or family member—opinions that are rarely based on anything concrete. Just because your friend had her bowel surgery done by Dr. Smith doesn't mean that Dr. Jones wouldn't do just as good a job. Just because I went to medical school with Dr. Pink doesn't mean that he'll treat you better than Dr. Green will. And in fact, if I'm honest, while I know Dr. Pink and believe him to be an intelligent person and a nice guy, I have no idea if his patients' outcomes are any better—or worse—than those of Dr. Green's patients. If a patient waiting for surgery wants to be seen by the surgeon with the lowest infection rates or the highest patient satisfaction ratings, fair enough. But that information is rarely publicly available in Canada. For patients who prefer to wait for a particular specialist, a longer wait may be worth it. But for many of us—myself included—being seen by a competent, well-trained professional as quickly as possible is the priority.

Centralized intake won't fix all the wait lists in Canada. But combined with other reforms, it would have a major impact. In particular, once a single common queue is implemented, we can begin to maximize the contributions of other, non-physician professionals to bring wait times down and improve the patient experience of care without spending more money.

2. Broaden Our Horizons

It can be easy to fall into the trap of thinking that health care is about doctors. But if we made better use of the tremendous expertise of other health care providers—and of the non-clinical staff in our health care organizations—we could go a long way toward delivering on the Triple Aim.

Centralized intake and assessment for hip and knee surgery is just one example. Too often, surgeon time is the bottleneck that causes the wait list to grow. But a nurse, nurse practitioner, physiotherapist, or pharmacist can do many of the tasks traditionally done by physicians (and often better than we can). Whether it's assessing patients' appropriateness for surgery or explaining to them how to start insulin or seeing them for a follow-up on their blood pressure, non-physicians can lead terrific models of care delivery.

You might be seen by a physician assistant in the emergency department or a nurse educator in a cancer clinic. You might get your primary care from a nurse practitioner. Your pharmacist might prescribe your medication renewal for you. In many cases this means that the care of a non-physician provider will *replace* at least part of what the doctor used to do rather than being *added* to that care, unless there is good evidence that the extra care provides better health outcomes and a better experience for the patient. In that case we may decide that the additional cost is acceptable. The concept of substituting rather than adding care will require teams to build deep trust and partnerships, but it's the only way we can improve the system at a cost we can all afford.

3. Use Hospitals Wisely

Every health care system needs hospitals. If I get hit by a car, or need my appendix taken out, or develop a life-threatening blood infection, I want to be taken to the hospital.

But much of what threatens our health doesn't kill us quickly, and it doesn't require big teams working on us around the clock. As the population ages and chronic disease rises, we should move care to where people need it: in their homes, or as close to their homes as possible. It's been said so many times that it feels almost trite to repeat it: the future of health is in primary care, home care, and self-care.

This doesn't mean that we should close hospitals or reduce the number of beds in Canada. We already have the lowest number of beds per capita among developed countries; the fat in Canadian hospitals was cut long ago. But we do need approaches that won't require us to massively increase the number of beds as the population ages. That's because the hospital is the most expensive part of the health care system, and because nobody wants to be there unless it's absolutely necessary.

And, of course, the front door to the hospital in Canada is the emergency department. Our EDs are the canaries in the coal mine: whether it's a backlog of patients on the ward waiting for long-term care or trouble accessing family doctors after hours, the ED is often where we see the first signs of trouble elsewhere in the system.

There are alternatives to hospitals and the ED. Michael Decter, the former deputy health minister I quoted earlier, has referred to the "six components of the out-of-hospital universe": primary health care, home care, the community pharmacy, community-based paramedicine or ambulance care, palliative care, and rehabilitation. Informal caregiving could be added to that list. And when patients with complex problems require more than what these seven out-of-hospital environments currently offer, we need better options than sending them to the emergency department or admitting (and readmitting, and re-readmitting) them to hospital.

Let's come back to Susan. If her family doctor—or one of his colleagues—had been available that winter morning when she started to feel weak, she might have gone to see him instead of going to the ED. Had she gone early enough, hopefully he could have given her advice that would help her get better at home. But what if she had arrived dehydrated and weak, clearly in need of IV rehydration? One look at her and the family doctor would have had no other option but to call 911 himself. In most communities there is no easy way to set up investigations and treatments in a timely manner outside the ED.

After Susan developed heart failure, every few months she landed back in the ED and was readmitted to hospital to deal with her chronic condition. That's an expensive and unpleasant way to manage exacerbations of chronic illness that are entirely predictable. We don't always know when they'll happen, but we know they will.

If Susan and her family doctor could have accessed specialty advice, urgent blood tests, X-ray exams, and IV treatments without having to call 911 every time she had such an exacerbation, her care would have been much better. If they could have accessed more intensive home supports for her, she might not have ended up sitting in hospital for weeks waiting for a long-term care bed.

Our downtown Toronto neighbourhood encompasses many family doctors like Susan's physician. They're solo practitioners, or they work in small groups of two or three doctors. They have large **practices, some**-times culturally or linguistically based, often Chinese- or **Portuguese**-speaking like many of my neighbours. They have many older patients who don't speak English well and who have complex medical needs. And they can often be fairly isolated from other services.

Like many Canadian emergency departments, the local ED is over-loaded, especially in the evenings and on weekends. And it's clear that gaps in communication and coordination with family doctors have resulted in fractured care and longer wait times for patients like Susan.

So a team of creative people led by two brilliant and brave women—Drs. Pauline Pariser and Gillian Hawker—set about to see how they could help. They launched a project called SCOPE (Seamless Care Opti-mizing the Patient Experience), which aims to help those family doctors in our neighbourhood keep patients like Susan *out* of the ED and prevent hospital admission when possible. This is all part of the mandate of Women's College Hospital as the "hospital to keep people out of hospital."

The target group of family doctors was identified through a method known as *hot-spotting*. The team looked at frequent flyers among the patients in the local emergency department and identified their family physicians. Solo doctors whose practices had high ED usage rates were offered the chance to join SCOPE.

Family doctors enrolled in SCOPE are provided with a "one number to call" service that helps them access advice from specialist doctors, gives them rapid access to urgent imaging for their patients, and assists with home care coordination. It also links them to the Acute Ambulatory Care Unit at Women's College Hospital.

The AACU is located where you'd expect to find the emergency department in a regular hospital, but it doesn't have a jam-packed wait-ing room or stretchers in the hallways. Instead, it's a calm place. On a busy day all the stretchers and rooms may be full, but people are flowing in and out of it the way they do through a clinic space. It isn't a walk-in service. Many patients who come to the AACU have done so because their family doctor is participating in the SCOPE project.

If Susan had gone to her family doctor's office right at the beginning of a mild exacerbation of her heart failure, he could have tinkered with her medications so that over the ensuing few days she'd pee away the extra fluid accumulating in her lungs. But for more severe symptoms, the only way to get her through would have been to give her IV medication and monitor her for a few hours—and there wouldn't have been anywhere for her to go other than the emergency department. She might spend several hours waiting there, and then another ten hours getting stabilized before being sent home. Or she might have been admitted to the hospital for a day or two. The routine would have always been the same: some blood work, a chest X-ray, some IV medications, and monitoring.

But if Susan's family doctor had been part of SCOPE, he would have had an alternative for her. He could have phoned the internal medicine specialist in the AACU on what I call the "magic cell phone"—magic because it's *answered!* by a *doctor!*—and that person would have told him to send her over. She wouldn't have had to wait. They'd have been expecting her, and the AACU doctor would have known what she needed because he'd have had a phone conversation with her family doctor. The AACU doctor and staff could have gotten a chest X-ray rapidly, given her some IV medicine, monitored her, and then sent her home with a connection to a home-care worker who could have checked on her the following day. Susan would have been well taken care of, and the experience would have been so much more pleasant. And the potential savings to the health system would have been significant, especially if a hospital admission had been avoided.

Patients like Susan aren't the only ones who can benefit from this model. One December, a woman whose family doctor was participating in SCOPE started experiencing severe pain in her bones. Blood tests revealed that she was developing kidney problems. She was given an appointment with a kidney specialist—a nephrologist—in mid-January. But by December 23 she'd become immobile. She was very frightened.

Instead of sending her to the ED, where she'd almost certainly have been admitted to hospital for a number of days over the busy holiday season, her family doctor arranged for her to be seen in the AACU at Women's College Hospital the next morning. She was there for six hours. She had a chest X-ray, an ultrasound, and a series of blood and urine tests. A pharmacist took a full history of her medications. She was examined by an internal medicine doctor. She was given a set of signs to watch for so that she'd know when to seek further medical attention, and was sent home with a short-term plan. Some of the blood work took time for the results to come back, so she returned two weeks later. A nurse practitioner went over all the results with her.

It wasn't until she met with the nephrologist in mid-January that she fully understood what SCOPE had done for her. Instead of having to send her for the many tests after meeting her, he already had all the results in front of him. With all that data, he was able to give her a diagnosis of probable (confirmed later) multiple myeloma—bone marrow cancer. It was not a happy diagnosis to receive, but she was glad to finally have all the pieces put together and to get on with the treatment plan.

We used to talk about "wrapping services around the patient." I never understood what that meant. As far as I could tell, it often seemed to mean throwing more and more health care at people: case workers, system navigators, specialized clinics for one body part or another. The SCOPE project instead wraps services around the primary care provider, helping family doctors take better care of complex patients in the community, close to home. New buildings and fancy technology aren't needed. What's needed is a willingness on the part of hospitals to organize their care differently, supporting primary care and home care workers who need backup. That way, patients can stay home instead of lying on stretchers in the emergency department or being admitted to hospital. SCOPE is one promising example, and others are emerging in communities across the country.

Of course, SCOPE is primarily about helping patients who need face-to-face care fairly quickly. But many elements of health care actually don't require that at all. This is where technology comes in.

4. Get Disruptive

Technology and virtual ways of providing care have the potential to transform health care, but not if we just layer them on top of our existing systems.

Disruptive technology offers products or services that are cheaper, simpler, or more convenient than the traditional way of doing things. What makes it disruptive is the fact that a smaller company or entity with fewer resources can successfully challenge the established order. Disruption happens when a new approach targets a group that has been overlooked, gaining a foothold by doing things in a way that's more attractive to consumers, often at a lower price.

Rather than focusing on small, incremental improvements to existing technology (like moving from a giant desktop computer to a slightly smaller desktop computer), disruptive innovation looks to find new approaches to tackling old challenges (like inventing the tablet). Early versions of disruptive technology often can't do as much as the traditional "gold standard" technology, just as the first laptops didn't have the computing power of a desktop. In health care these are often "good enough" approaches to care that gain acceptance, improve, and sometimes even go on to destroy the market for much more expensive and traditional approaches. Whether it's a finger prick blood test for HIV that's slightly less accurate but can be administered anywhere, including in a small rural clinic, or the deployment of more easily trained health care providers to perform tasks that used to be performed by doctors, disruptive innovations push the boundaries of our established ways of doing things and lower the price of care.

One night when I was working in the emergency department in a small northern Ontario community, a young girl was brought into the ED by her distraught grandmother. Her family lived in rudimentary housing on a nearby Aboriginal reserve. The temperature control on the water tank hadn't been working for months and they couldn't get it fixed, so if the hot water tap was turned on, the water came out scalding hot. The grandmother was taking care of the kids. While she was tending to the baby, the little girl turned the kitchen tap on with her feet dangling in the sink. She suffered immediate severe burns on both legs.

The traditional approach to caring for this child would have been to fly her and one family member hundreds of kilometres away to the nearest pediatric burn centre for weeks of monitoring and daily dressing changes. Instead, we called on the Ontario Telemedicine Network. OTN connects patients with a care team in a major centre through the use of video communication.

We admitted that little girl to our small rural hospital and immediately got onto a video call with a burn specialist. She evaluated the size and severity of the burns and helped us figure out how best to dress them, how much fluid to give the patient, and which antibiotics to give her. She continued to assess those burns every day through remote video-conferencing. The patient was able to stay where her whole family could be with her. The system was saved the costs of travel, family accommodation, and a stay in a tertiary care hospital. That was my first contact with disruptive technology in health care, and I was amazed.

It seemed futuristic and far-fetched at the time—this was the early 2000s—but telemedicine has now become normal across rural communities in many parts of Canada. And it works. For example, during a three-year research trial, a stroke rehabilitation program conducted through telemedicine rather than traditional face-to-face visits demonstrated no difference in treatment outcomes. I suspect that in the early days, a cardiologist listening to someone's heart through video technology would have said it was "good enough" but not as good as laying hands on the patient. And maybe a psychotic patient being assessed by a psychiatrist through technology would prefer to be in the same room as the doctor asking all those personal questions. But the increased convenience, equivalent health outcomes, and lower cost make virtual care the kind of disruptive technology we need to pursue. We can give tablets to providers in big hospitals so that they can walk around and take notes as they go, and that may represent a process improvement—but it isn't disruptive. It's just layering technology on top of the existing system. We need to seek disruption.

5. Help People Die with Dignity

Sometimes it makes sense to use everything within our powers to try and cure or interrupt the progression of illness. But at other times those efforts merely reduce patients' quality of life for the valuable, limited time they have left. People who are not physically strong may not be able to benefit from, or even handle, intense treatments. So whereas traditional therapeutic care strives to get resolution to health problems, palliative care seeks to control or eliminate *symptoms* in order that we can live well for as long as we have. And that can be a long time! The transition to a palliative set of goals doesn't always mean that the patient will die immediately. It does mean that the goals of treatment change, which, if the process is managed well, can be a relief for patients, families, and their care teams.

Still, our palliative care systems in Canada have traditionally been focused on care at the very end of life. Instead of encouraging an early connection for those with incurable illness and providing support for a longer period of time, many of these programs and services have eligibility criteria that require a prognosis of less than three months. The result is that people often spend their final year or years of life bouncing in and out of hospital, receiving treatments that aren't benefiting them, before finally being transitioned to palliative care that would have helped them cope well with their situation sooner. For most people, there isn't a single moment when it becomes suddenly clear that we need to shift from a curative to a palliative framework. Instead, doctors and patients can slowly shift the orientation away from more invasive tests and procedures and toward a broader focus on quality of life. Too often, we don't have reliable systems in place to help people through that process.

With an aging population and the advanced chronic illness it can bring, we desperately need new approaches to dealing with illness that can't be cured. These approaches must respect what frail patients and their families want. Palliative care is not about hastening the end of life or denying people cures. It's about helping patients decide what they want by having a realistic conversation about their options.

The PATH clinic in Nova Scotia is one place where that conversation is occurring. PATH is essentially a program that helps older people and their families plan. Through guided conversations, decision aids, and education, seniors can better understand their health status, anticipate what lies ahead for them, and learn what they can do about it; in short, the program enables them to navigate through the process of making health care decisions. PATH also offers training for health care teams so that they can improve the quality of those conversations.

For older people with serious health conditions, including those who have one or more advanced or progressive illnesses and have been in and out of hospital, a process like this is critically needed. It would have been a great program for Susan when she was in her last year of life and kept being admitted to the hospital.

Eventually, the end comes for us all. Although most Canadians want to die either at home or in some other safe, comfortable, non-hospital setting, more than half of all deaths occur in hospital. As we've seen, hard-wired patterns across our systems mean that patients, particularly older adults, are shipped to acute care—from home or a long-term care facility—when they're very ill, even when these patients and their providers have agreed that curative care is not the preferred way to go. So if we really want to support Canadians in dying where they want to die—which is usually not in acute care hospitals—we're going to need to scale up successful models of home palliative care.

In recent years, our palliative systems have been very focused on cancer. Yet there is a growing recognition that too many patients with chronic conditions for which we don't have cures—such as end-stage lung disease, and the heart failure that Susan had—do not yet have adequate access to palliative and end-of-life care. For those who do, their care is far superior.

When I was a trainee in the hospital setting, we'd always ask older people with chronic conditions whether they'd want to be resuscitated if their heart stopped beating or they stopped breathing while they were in hospital. Did they want tubes put down their throats? Shocks administered to their chests? Did they want to be hooked up to a breathing machine?

We rarely sat down and asked them how they wanted to spend whatever time they might have left and how we could help them achieve those goals. That's the conversation we all deserve to have if we're lucky to live long enough. Yes, we're back to focusing on relationships as the core of positive patient experience.

————

The notion of partnering more deeply with patients is surfacing all over the health care system. Barbara Balik, a health care leader in the U.K., has nicely summarized this by noting that countries have been slowly evolving from providing care "to patients" to providing it "for patients" to providing it "with patients."

Redesign of health care delivery, if done in true partnership with the people who use the system, can achieve the Triple Aim. We can reduce wait times by reorganizing processes of care; we can offer people with chronic illness alternatives to treatment in the ED and dying in hospital; we can introduce technology in exciting ways that will improve value in the system. And we can do all that without infusing more money into it. But in order to know how to design programs that achieve those goals, patients need to be involved from the start. It's the patients who'll tell us where the system's fault lines are and help us design better approaches. They'll also help us evaluate our new models by telling us how to measure what matters to them.

Patient experience—one of the three prongs of the Triple Aim—is about how people experience their own care and the care of their loved ones as they go through the system. But patient *engagement* extends beyond involvement at the individual level. Making decisions about the ways we organize care, especially when those new models challenge the status quo and require a culture shift, should be done with citizens—not just communicated to them after the fact.

Consider the Northumberland Hills Hospital in the town of Cobourg, Ontario, which faced difficult choices during its 2010 fiscal year. The 110-bed hospital had run operating deficits for three years in order to maintain the twenty-three services that its community had come to expect. Instead of making tough decisions and then trying to explain them publicly, the NHH board embarked on a public consultation about how to balance its budget. In that small community, heavily invested in its hospital as both an employer and a provider of services, the board struck a Citizens' Advisory Panel of randomly selected people. Panel members got a crash course in the hospital: over a period of ten months, they toured the wards; heard from experts, stakeholders, and service providers; and talked to their neighbours. They hosted town hall meetings. They deliberated. Eventually they brought recommendations to the hospital board about how to balance its budget. This meant making some hard calls, like closing programs, but the decisions were made based on the community's priorities.

Of course, as we begin to implement system solutions that allow us to do more with less, a good number of our terrific ideas won't pan out. What do we do when that happens?

The F-Word

Failure. The converging currents of an aging population, a rise in complex chronic illness, a desire to move care out of hospitals and into the community, and a pressure to curtail rising costs all mean that we have to try new things in health care. And if we're being sufficiently innovative, a lot of them won't work.

As any entrepreneur will tell you, innovation is a risky business. We used to say 50 percent of startups fail; research now suggests that number is over 90 percent. In the business world, it sometimes seems as though people wear their failures as badges of honour—since, after all, failure is the flip side of innovation. The famous management consultant John Maxwell even wrote a whole book called *Failing Forward*. And what's true in life and in business is also true in health care: if we're not failing, we aren't stretching ourselves sufficiently.

Fear of failure has held us back from implementing the kinds of innovative delivery models we need, and from evaluating those models when we do implement them. What hospital wants to discover that its new diabetes program doesn't improve outcomes in diabetics? What primary care team wants to know that its new online appointment-booking approach is worse than the old phone system? What minister of health wants to stand up in Question Period and defend the investment that yielded nothing better than what we had before?

Several years ago, Dr. Irfan Dhalla and his team designed the "Virtual Ward," a program targeted at patients who were being discharged from hospital but were known to be at high risk of readmission. The Virtual Ward provided patients with all the elements of a hospital ward—doctors, nurses, pharmacists, daily rounds, ready access to tests and treatments—but in their own home. It was intended for patients like Susan, who have complex medical issues and are frequently being admitted and readmitted to hospital.

The Virtual Ward was the first project in Ontario to articulate, design, and rigorously test a new model like this. The Ministry of Health had the courage and good sense to fund the study and wait for the results instead of just implementing this terrific idea across the health care system. It was a victory of science over intuitive policy making.

Yet, despite the project's great potential, the results of the evaluation were disappointing. The providers involved felt that the Virtual Ward improved the quality of care for complex patients after they were discharged, particularly those who were homebound or without access to primary care. But the primary outcomes for Virtual Ward patients— readmission to the hospital and death—did not significantly differ from those who received "usual care."

We know this because the team had the fortitude to rigorously evaluate it. No harm was done to the patients of the Virtual Ward. The team at Women's College Hospital that ran the program survived the disappointment and applied what they'd learned to subsequent projects. Too often new programs are put in place in health care without any such evaluation. We try something because the innovation sounds good—but we don't collect any data to determine whether it actually does good.

Publicly accountable institutions can be very risk averse, and understandably so. Leaders and health care providers fear litigation or humiliation if something new doesn't work, so they may stick with something old . . . even if we already know that it doesn't work. But as we tackle new ways of delivering health care, we need to think about how we can learn from failure rather than running from it. And in that, we have much to learn from our colleagues in the private sector.

According to the business literature, an organization must do two things to succeed: execute and innovate. Therefore, there are two kinds of failure. The first is failure in *execution*. We know what needs to be done, but we fail to do it consistently. For example, when we know what best practice looks like yet we still see big variations in care across a region, that represents an execution failure.

We're slowly shifting the culture of health care—moving from sweeping failures under the rug to collectively learning from our shortcomings. Instead of blaming individual providers when we fall short of best practice, health care organizations are beginning to build systems to support learning and improvement. For example, we know that many patients acquire infections while in hospital because health care workers don't consistently wash their hands before and after touching people and surfaces, thus transmitting infections from one patient to another. So we're increasingly monitoring handwashing rates and infection rates in Canadian hospitals, and reporting those rates publicly. Publicizing these kinds of execution failures can create pressure to improve. Departments hold competitions to reduce their infection rates. Handwashing stations are placed prominently outside every patient room. Patients and family members are encouraged to ask their providers whether they've washed their hands or to fill out questionnaires about whether the doctor or nurse did so before performing a procedure. In short, monitoring and reporting—as our provincial Health Quality Councils often compel us to do—are part of the solution to execution failures, because they force us to strive to do better when we actually know what "better" looks like.

The second kind of failure is the failure to *search for innovation* when there are many unknowns. For example, when we're faced with an aging population with changing needs and yet continue to operate in the same old way, that represents an innovation failure.

This problem is harder to solve. Innovation initiatives can't be held to the same standard as those of existing products. When creativity and risk king are required, we need different processes, procedures, schedules, and incentives to allow innovation in health care delivery to thrive. Searching for new ways of doing things means accepting a higher degree of risk than we're accustomed to.

I became interested in failure when my friend Alissa sent me a link to the first Failure Report I'd ever seen. Engineers Without Borders sends engineers to developing countries to build bridges, dig wells, and design critical infrastructure. It's hard to imagine work more important, so you'd think the organization would be pretty focused on success. But every year, along with reporting its achievements, EWB publishes a Failure Report. These reports do more than just acknowledge failure—they openly celebrate it. The EWB leaders accept the notion that to be a high-performing innovation organization you need to take risks, which means that some of your projects will fail. By publicizing and trying to learn from each failed project, EWB sets the standard for how those of us working in life-or-death situations can approach our own challenges.

The prospect may make some people feel uncomfortable. How could we *celebrate* failure in health care? When we put hundreds of thousands of dollars into a project to try to lower the rate of hospital admissions through a Virtual Ward and it doesn't work, haven't we just wasted tax dollars and potentially harmed people? Surely learning from these experiences doesn't require celebrating them.

I think it should. I'm in favour of celebrating failure and scaling it up—so that any unsuccessful health care project is widely publicized and the reasons for its failure are discussed openly across the system. This doesn't mean we take the consequences lightly. But if we deem a risk worth taking, we need to honour the work and innovation that went into it and the lessons we've learned.

So how do we create a health system that responds usefully to failure and supports learning from it?

As Dr. Joshua Tepper, the CEO of Health Quality Ontario, has said, part of what we need to do is make the declaration of failure a routine part of our work—just as EWB does by publishing its annual Failure Report. Finding ways to share failures across the system can't be left to individual brave organizations; the first to take that courageous step risks being crucified in the media or in Question Period. Particularly in a publicly funded health care system where elected politicians are held accountable for the performance of our health and social services, exposing failure is often left to journalists and auditors general rather than careful self-reflection. We tend to design our reporting in order to highlight successes—to declare victory as quickly as possible—rather than to drive improvements. By making the declaration and analysis of failure routine, we can begin to turn this around. Organizations like Health Quality Councils have a huge role to play in this kind of reporting, because they can supply the mechanisms to do it in ways that emphasize learning rather than blame.

The other thing we need to do is resist the temptation to deal with failure in a black and white way. Too often in health care we either continue failed projects or toss them in the garbage bin entirely. The problem is that both responses show an absence of thoughtful adaptation. If we don't actually internalize the lessons from failure, we can't possibly hope to succeed.

Which brings me back to the Virtual Ward project. It was set up as a randomized controlled trial, and it took fully three years to conclude that its design wasn't the right one to reduce hospital readmissions. The tried-and-true scientific approach to testing a new model of medical care is, after all, a very methodical process. Each step occurs in sequence: designing the solution, implementing it, verifying its implementation, and then maintaining it. There is a long process of collecting data, followed by an analysis to determine whether the intervention led to a better outcome for people than the usual way of doing things.

But as Virtual Ward demonstrated, you can spend a lot of time developing something that ends up not working. This traditional scientific approach doesn't allow for modifications based on what's learned during implementation. For example, say you're trying to test the effectiveness of a new diabetes education program that helps diabetics learn about nutrition. About halfway through, it becomes clear that your participants need and want more support than just education. They need help, for instance, with transportation to get to a grocery store with more affordable healthy food. But at this point you can't change your intervention because it would skew the results of your study.

So the Virtual Ward team and other project teams at the Women's College Hospital Institute for Health System Solutions and Virtual Care are now taking a different approach. Instead of designing large-scale classical research trials, they're engaging in Silicon Valley thinking, making frequent and rapid changes to the design of their projects. Based on what they learn almost weekly, they can make changes and measure the impact again and again in order to build models of care that don't just sound good, but actually work. Rather than continuing to execute a promising but flawed concept or taking months or years to test an updated version that's set in stone, they've learned to "pivot": to rapidly change the programs in response to new information on how best to achieve their overarching goal. They try changing which patients they target. They try making the health care team smaller or larger. They try educating patients directly instead of giving information to their family doctors. And with each pivot, projects like the Virtual Ward can come closer to a model that's able to effectively deliver on its objective.

———

As a respected friend and mentor said to me about the concept of doing more with less, the million-dollar question in all of this is to figure out how to rebuild the plane while it's flying. How do we reorganize and free up resources to improve care delivery while people like Susan still keep showing up in hospital?

If we think about our challenge as the need to both execute and innovate at the same time, we can find our way through. When we fail to execute (as evidenced in the problem of regional variations in care), we need to identify successful models—also known as positive outliers—and spread and scale them.

But in other cases we face complex problems, great uncertainty, and no clear solutions. Our risk there isn't execution failure, but rather failure to search for innovation. And the culture that can respond to that challenge is startup culture. Groups trying new ways of delivering care that fail fast, adapt quickly, and know how to execute rapid experimentation—like the Virtual Ward leaders—are essentially running what the business world calls "lean startups." These are small groups that prioritize experimentation over exhaustive planning and that value patient and provider feedback over intuition. Instead of planning big projects for a long time, they experiment rapidly and on a small scale, trying different things, checking whether they work, tweaking their design, and trying again. This approach to redesign involves heavy evaluation, but it isn't traditional research. It involves Silicon Valley thinking, but it isn't for profit.

There are proven ways for payers, like governments, to promote experimentation and innovation while still keeping the plane flying. They can carve out space in our organizations for innovation, encouraging teams to break the rules and think differently about evaluation. That process is unfolding all around us; it's an exciting time to be involved in Canadian health care reform. Money is likely to be tight for the foreseeable future, but more money probably wouldn't buy us what we need anyway. What we need is to channel our creativity to do things differently, with clear goals to improve not only the health of our patients but also their experience of care—for no more money than we already spend.

By reorganizing the delivery of services in ways that respect both the people who work in the system and the people who need care, we really can do more with less. If we let go of some traditions, if we centralize intake for specialty services and help our non-physician providers work to the full scope of their skills, and if we use technology in unexpected ways to direct people with chronic disease away from the emergency department, we'll make much better use of our resources. Supporting people at the end of life in a manner that honours their wishes and welcoming patient input in our design process will result in a more humane system. Along the way, we're sure to use the F-word—failure—but it's time to take that risk.

BIG IDEA 5

LESLIE: BASIC INCOME FOR BASIC HEALTH

Sick with Poverty

Nothing makes health care providers feel more powerless than being confronted with a patient whose poor health we can't improve. In my practice, it's patients like Leslie who often remind me of the limits of my usefulness.

Leslie is a single mom who used to live in downtown Toronto. I've been her family doctor for a decade. When I met her, she was living with her teenaged son and was in close daily contact with her father. She had her share of health problems, but they didn't stop her from living her life. Then her breathing troubles began.

Leslie suffers from severe asthma. She uses multiple puffers and has been on and off prednisone (a powerful drug with significant side effects) many times to try to control her symptoms. She's been seen by specialists and has been in and out of the emergency department dozens of times.

But she didn't have asthma when I met her. It started when the social housing unit she lived in had a flood. Mould grew inside the walls of the building, and Leslie's health began to deteriorate. She took photos of the mould and brought them to her landlord. Her doctors, including me, wrote letters of support, trying to get her moved to another apartment or another building.

During that time, her physical and mental health deteriorated. She became depressed. Her relationships fell apart. She gained weight and her blood pressure worsened, in part because she couldn't exercise due to her breathing problems.

And it seemed to her that all she did was cough. She was up much of the night coughing, and felt terrible because she kept her son up. She was afraid to take the subway to come to my office because she felt that people were staring at her; she felt compelled to explain to strangers everywhere she went that her cough wasn't contagious. Sometimes she'd cough so hard that she'd lose control of her bladder. That happened once in a public place, and she stopped wanting to go out.

I referred her to a lung specialist, who patiently explained to Leslie that her cough wouldn't resolve itself until she got out of her apartment. But Leslie didn't have anywhere else to go. She stayed, and fought to be transferred to a different housing unit.

There was a period of time when seeing Leslie's name on my clinic list meant preparing myself to write letters or fill out forms, and lots of them. Letters to the social housing authority, to her building super-intendent, to her case worker. Forms for social assistance money for transportation to and from her many medical appointments. And then, as it became clear that her health wasn't going to improve, appli-cation forms for permanent disability benefits. Her life was a maze of bureaucracy.

It took her, and us, two years to get the system to respond to her requests for a new apartment in Toronto's social housing system. By the time she moved, to an apartment far from her existing community, she wasn't the same person anymore.

On the bright side, her cough has improved substantially in the years since she left. But there's a zest missing in her. Every time I see Leslie, I revisit a feeling of helplessness and shame that I wasn't able to do more to help.

There's a reason I felt powerless in the face of Leslie's cough. As my colleague Dr. Ryan Meili, an expert in the root causes of illness, would say, Leslie wasn't sick with asthma. She was sick with poverty—and she still is. She wasn't struck down with cancer; she was afflicted by a lack of access to appropriate housing and the basic human dignity that comes with being able to make the choices we all want to make to stay healthy. One of the best ways to help Leslie and other Canadians facing the same challenges can be explained without even a passing reference to health care. But acting on it would do more to improve health than any single other policy our governments could embrace.

Far more than consumption of medical care, income is the strongest predictor of health. Canadians are more likely to die at an earlier age and suffer more illnesses if they are in a low income bracket, regardless of age, sex, race, and place of residence.

There are at least two ways in which income is related to health. First, income allows people to purchase the things that are necessary to survive and thrive, such as nutritious food and safe shelter. Second, income affects health indirectly, through its effect on social participation and the ability to control life circumstances. Poverty limits people's choices in their social networks, the jobs they can access, and their sense of control over their own destinies.

Put another way, the biggest disease that needs to be cured in Canada is the disease of poverty. And part of the cure is to implement the fifth Big Idea: A Basic Income Guarantee for all Canadians.

———

There's an old parable that's often used to illustrate the importance of looking "upstream" to understand what makes people sick and so address the root causes of illness.

> You are standing on the edge of a river. All of a sudden a flailing, drowning child comes floating by. Without thinking, you dive in, grab the child, and swim to shore. Before you can recover, another child comes floating by, so you dive in and rescue her as well. Then another child drifts into sight, and another and another. Everyone standing on the shore is diving into the water to rescue them.

Eventually, some wise person will ask: "Why do these kids keep falling into the river?" And they'll head upstream to find out.

Decades of studies have demonstrated that, as important as health care is, it doesn't play the primary role in determining whether people will be ill or well. Social and economic factors—*upstream* factors like those that led to Leslie's illness—have a much more powerful impact on the most meaningful outcomes. These factors are referred to as "the social determinants of health." If addressed, they can have a profound effect on the health of both individuals and communities. Tackling them amounts to building a fence at the top of the river to prevent children from falling into the water.

Although health care currently takes up nearly half of provincial budgets and is consistently ranked as a top priority for Canadians, health care systems determine only 25 percent of the health of populations. Our social and economic environments account for fully half of the health of a population.

The social determinants of health include things like income, housing, education, food security, Aboriginal status, gender, and race. Leslie's case, for example, illustrates how housing can affect health. But to separate the social determinants from one another is to miss how interrelated they are. They intermingle and interact with each other in so many complex ways. Poverty leads to lower educational attainment—and vice versa—which limits people's job prospects, which are also narrowed by racism, which in turn leads to chronic stress and illness, which makes it hard to keep a full-time job, which leads to worse poverty. The social determinants of health pile up, making it hard to escape a vicious cycle that inevitably leads to, among other things, poor health.

Of course, deciding whether to fish drowning children out of the water or look upstream to figure out why they keep falling in is a false choice. We need to do both. A strong, equitably designed health care system is one of the best ways to mitigate the effects of social inequality. But if all we do is pour money into the child-saving brigade rather than building fences around the top of the river, we'll be fighting a losing battle. In particular, if we want to address the social determinants of health in Canada, we need to put an end to Canada's biggest killer: poverty.

———

The case for the elimination of poverty on health grounds is compelling. If we were to choose only one social determinant on which to focus our attention, it should be poverty. It has the biggest impact on health of any determinant, and it's a major problem in Canada.

Poverty has an effect on health that crosses generations. The children of low-income parents are in worse health than the children of higher income parents. The long-term outcomes of children from low-income families are also worse in terms of their ability to get good jobs and contribute to the economy. I see this in my daily work, including with Leslie's son, Darius, who has opted not to pursue any education beyond high school. This doesn't mean that he'll never have well-paid work, but his chances are hindered.

Differences in the health of children from high- and low-income families begin at birth, continue through life, and lead to differences in health in the children of children born into poverty. These differences are apparent in lower birth weights, higher rates of asthma and mental health conditions, and poorer vision, hearing, speech, and mobility. They're also reflected in levels of exposure to toxic chemicals, such as pollutants like second-hand smoke, and in the rates of accidents and injuries. Even in countries like Canada with universal health insurance, poor children are in worse health than richer children, and poor adults are in worse health than richer adults.

Understanding why low-income families might have children with more health problems in the short and long term helps us understand the effects of poverty on health more broadly. Kids like Darius don't lack for love or parental commitment to their well-being. But they have fewer opportunities to participate in organized activities and lessons, fewer educational resources at home, and in many cases, a significant degree of economic and psychological stress—particularly in single-parent households. Leslie's stress as a single parent struggling to make ends meet may have affected Darius's preparedness for learning when he was entering school, limiting his subsequent academic performance.

As they grow up, kids who did not overcome the barriers they faced earlier on in life may enter lower wage jobs and repeat the cycle of poverty with their own families.

They may move into low-cost housing in a neighbourhood like the south section of Point Douglas, Winnipeg, an area where male life expectancy is sixty-seven years, whereas in some of the city's wealthier neighbourhoods it's eighty-five. This is the part of the city with the highest number of homes in need of major repair and where pregnant women face double the city average of family risk factors for an unhealthy pregnancy, including alcohol or tobacco use, financial difficulties, and mental illness. Those kinds of risk factors affect not only the woman and her pregnancy, but also the future mental and intellectual development of the baby on the way.

———

We ought to care about the impact of poverty on health because we're a society that cares about human rights. We should also care because poverty is expensive for all of us. If you live in Ontario, poverty costs your household nearly $3000 per year in the form of increased costs to social systems and lost revenues to the province. In other provinces, the numbers are no better: the estimated cost of poverty in Saskatchewan alone is $3.8 billion per year.

About two-thirds of that cost comes from decreased economic activity, as 10 percent of the population isn't out there earning money and spending it. The other third comes from the increased health, social, and justice costs that result from lives led in poverty. Canadians who don't live in deep poverty are paying for those services and for lost contributions to the economy because so many of our neighbours can't make ends meet. The economic impact on each of us is significant.

Poverty isn't just bad for the health of poor people. When poverty is a serious problem and income inequality is high, the health of the entire population is affected, not just the health of the poor.

The question of inequality—how big the gap is between rich and poor—is an important one. Even if we can reduce the number of Canadians living below a certain income level, a growing gap between the highest and the lowest earners may still be of concern. There is a case—highly suggestive, although still being debated and explored— that reducing income inequality would benefit the health of the entire Canadian population.

In their book *The Spirit Level: Why Greater Equality Makes Societies Stronger*, Richard Wilkinson and Kate Pickett document how outcomes for eleven different health and social problems (including mental health, physical health, teenage pregnancies, drug abuse, and child well-being) are worse in wealthy countries where the gap between rich and poor is wider and better where it is narrower. If we want to improve health, we probably need to address not just absolute poverty but also inequality.

In Canada we often speak proudly of our social safety net, but the reality is that many of our "poverty reduction programs" are an exercise in scarcity and humiliation. I don't know how anyone survives on social assistance. For example, the current rate in Newfoundland for a couple with children, including a housing allowance, is around $1100 a month. But the average monthly rent for a two-bedroom apartment is $893 in St John's. How can we reasonably expect people to take care of themselves, eat decent food, and look for work if nearly every penny they receive goes toward rent? The problem reproduces itself in communities across Canada.

Even if we increased the amount of support provided to people on welfare, our systems remain highly bureaucratic and demoralizing for those who constantly have to prove they "deserve" support. As former senator Hugh Segal has pointed out, this is "deeply inefficient, fraught with bureaucratic excess and causes the wrong incentives to prevail." Life on social assistance is a labyrinth of case workers, forms, claims denials, and self-justification. This system feels designed to limit access as much as possible, not to ensure that all those who need support actually get it.

As Leslie tried to navigate our systems of welfare and disability, it often seemed to me that her full-time job was satisfying the requirements of the system that was supposed to be helping her. The rules can be stifling: literally hundreds of them govern each of our social assistance programs, all of them requiring time, energy, and money to police. Case workers in the welfare system work hard and surely believe in the importance of compassion and respect, but they operate in a system that can make it difficult to deliver on those principles.

People on social assistance also often experience what is known as the "welfare wall": it can be worse for them to work than not to work. This is because, in a number of provincial welfare regimes, coming off assistance means losing their drug coverage and other benefits. Furthermore, assistance is clawed back if they earn any income at all—and if they get a job and then lose it, the whole bureaucratic process of applying for assistance starts all over again.

For many, the application process and the constant negotiations are frustrating and feel unfair. A case worker's discretion can make the difference between getting what others in their situation receive and not getting anything at all. Moreover, if a mother finds a job for minimum wage, we suspend dental or drug care benefits for both her *and* her children. We also cut off support to people if they apply for a student loan—even though an education is their best chance of getting out of poverty. If this seems counterintuitive, it's because it is. Segal sums it up nicely: "Our present system does not fight poverty. It institutionalizes it."

Curing Income Deficiency

Poverty is a complex social problem, with ongoing debate even about how to define it. But at its core is a simple reality: people living in poverty have a deficiency of income. We can eliminate income poverty by ensuring that no one in Canada has an income below what's needed to achieve a basic standard of living. If we did so, we'd see a considerable improvement in the health of Canadians.

The Basic Income Guarantee is a well-developed approach to reducing poverty. It goes by various names (such as the guaranteed annual income, the negative income tax, and the basic income), and there are different ways to design it. The version I like best works like this: if your income from all sources falls below a certain level, you get topped up to a level sufficient to meet basic needs. That's it.

A true Basic Income Guarantee would ensure that everyone in Canada has an income above the "poverty line." In other words, it would virtually eliminate poverty in Canada.

This approach differs from costly and bureaucratic social assistance programs in two critical ways. First, social assistance in Canada tends to provide a level of support well below the poverty line. Second, because it would work through the tax system, the Basic Income Guarantee would eliminate complex eligibility and exemption criteria, making it quite administratively simple. The *only* criterion for eligibility would be a person's level of income. It wouldn't matter who you live with or whether you search for work or attend a training program.

One of the original fans of the Basic Income Guarantee was, believe it or not, the famous libertarian economist Milton Friedman—the man who inspired Ronald Reagan's economic policies. Friedman envisioned a world in which all other forms of social welfare would be abolished, a pretty extreme view that's hard to imagine today. The Basic Income Guarantee can't and mustn't replace all social programs. We still need good public education, publicly financed health care, quality affordable child care, affordable housing, and reliable unemployment insurance (policies that Friedman argued against). But Friedman was right that a system that puts money in people's pockets based on their take-home income is more cost-effective and more administratively efficient than one that requires them to prove how worthy they are in a hundred other ways.

What makes the Basic Income Guarantee attractive is that it would eliminate the need for the kinds of income support programs that invade people's lives and limit their choices. Many existing programs, such as social assistance in Canada or food stamp programs in the United States, are based on a highly paternalistic approach to social welfare. Such systems also require substantial administrative investments—forms have to be filled out, case workers must meet with recipients (sometimes going to their homes to ascertain that the rules are being honoured), people are required to prove that they've been looking for work and to account for how they spend their money . . . the list goes on. So it's no wonder that the fiscally conservative and the socially liberal alike support the notion that grown people shouldn't be policed in their consumption and that paternalistic systems of welfare are a waste of money.

No Canadian has expressed the benefits of the Basic Income Guarantee better than former Conservative senator Hugh Segal. As he's consistently pointed out, if our tax system topped up everyone who was beneath the poverty line to above it, we'd liberate millions of dollars currently used on provincial social assistance programs. And recipients "would not be treated as dim creatures, incapable of making decisions; they would be treated as human beings trusted to make life choices."

———

When I was a resident working at St. Michael's Hospital in Toronto, I followed a few women through the entirety of their pregnancies and births. It's an amazing experience to get to know someone just as she's beginning her pregnancy, to be there for the birth of that baby, and then to continue to follow the whole family as their family doctor.

One case left a mark on me for another reason. Fatou, a young woman who'd recently arrived in Canada from Senegal with no family or other supports, came under my care for her pregnancy. As a French-speaking immigrant she was happy to discover that I spoke French, and I felt from the outset that we had a bond. This was strengthened by the fact that I knew she had little support in the country, so I took my job as her family doctor, responsible for helping her through her pregnancy, very seriously.

As I began seeing Fatou for her regular prenatal checkups, I became very conscious of her vulnerability. She was a beautiful young woman who dressed in traditional fabrics, colourful prints that couldn't have kept her very warm through a Toronto winter. She spoke the lilting French of francophone Africa, which is similar to the French I grew up with and always strikes a chord in my heart.

I knew that Fatou was underhoused, moving back and forth between the homes of members of her community and a women's shelter, and that she was on social assistance. The funding rate for an individual adult on social assistance, even with the small pregnancy supplement, is not enough to live on in downtown Toronto.

We had long conversations about how to take care of herself in her pregnancy. We talked about healthy eating, plans for her living arrangements after the baby came, and what to expect at the hospital. I knew she'd need help getting by, so I gave her printouts with lists of public health dental clinics, local food banks, and charities that provided some basics to low-income new mothers. Proud of my awareness of the social determinants of health, I felt I was really doing right by her.

However, I became concerned in the middle of her second trimester: Fatou was simply not gaining weight. Her belly was getting bigger, but I could see that the rest of her was shrinking. I sent her for various tests looking for thyroid problems or parasites. Over and over I explained to her how much she had to eat in order to maintain a healthy pregnancy. I told her to make sure she went to the food bank if she couldn't afford to buy the food herself. I drew little maps of where the food bank was. I found myself feeling frustrated because I was working so hard to help her and felt she wasn't doing her part to help herself.

After weeks of these discussions, she finally broke down crying. She explained that she'd been going to the food bank, but that she'd had to throw out most of what she got there. It all came in weird boxes and she couldn't figure out what it was or how to prepare it. This was the food of the poor in North American society: boxes of macaroni and powdered cheese, cans of ravioli, and other items that were essentially unrecognizable to her as food. She didn't know what to do with it. And she was too ashamed to say so; instead, she went hungry. Had she been given a bag of rice and a bag of beans, Fatou would have known what to do. Better yet, if she'd been given the money she needed to live on, she could have purchased and prepared food herself.

I remember this case with shame. I did too much talking and not enough listening. I also remember it as a powerful illustration of how wrong we are as a society to think we know better than people themselves do about how to spend their money. When we try to micro-manage our assistance to people in order to prevent "waste" of collective resources, we insult their humanity and their intelligence. And we don't help them much at all.

———

Once we agree on the principle of the Basic Income Guarantee, the question is how to implement it. There are two major schools of thought.

The first supports the guaranteed annual income, also called a "negative income tax." In this model, everyone submits their tax returns to the government, and those who earn less than a set amount receive a top-up to bring them to that level. At a certain level of income, people wouldn't receive a subsidy but also wouldn't pay any taxes; above that level, the progressive income tax system would kick in, never allowing any one adult to fall below an after-tax minimum income. Households with more than one adult or with children would receive a larger benefit to reflect the reality of what's needed to meet their basic needs. The easiest way to think about this is to imagine that children, too, receive an income, and that it comes to them through their parents—although the income for a child would be less than for an adult.

The guaranteed annual income works like a refundable tax credit. Those who have no income from any other source would receive a basic entitlement. As the amount they earn increases, the benefit declines but less than proportionately—it isn't a dollar-for-dollar clawback on their earnings. Consequently, low-income earners receive partial benefits so that they're not worse off than they would be if they quit their jobs and relied only on the basic income. As a result there's always an incentive to work: people who work are always better off than they would be if they didn't work.

The second possible way to design a Basic Income Guarantee is as a universal cash transfer, also known as a "basic income" or a "demogrant." This is where a set amount of money is paid out to every individual in society, regardless of his or her income. This is how Old Age Security works in Canada: it's paid to all seniors at all income levels.

This design would involve the government issuing a cash transfer—enough to live on, or to substantially supplement the lowest income—to every single Canadian. Higher income earners would eventually pay much of it back in taxes, but the transfer would be paid out to everyone.

The notion of the universal cash transfer is attractive in some ways, particularly because universal programs tend to create a sense of social cohesion. They engender the support of wealthier citizens, who receive the transfer even though they'll pay taxes on it, and the structure removes any potential stigma associated with receiving the benefit. Again, Old Age Security is a great example of this.

A cash transfer of this kind would not be a small amount of money. It would be a "basic income"—enough to live on. Most versions that currently exist in other countries, such as the Brazilian Bolsa Família (Family Grant), are more income supplements than full basic incomes— but many countries have significant experience with modest cash transfers. In Brazil, the program electronically transfers monthly cash allowances to bank cards that are entrusted to the heads of households that qualify.

With the Bolsa Família, some very basic conditions apply—not the kinds of conditions we have for welfare, but instead mandatory prenatal care for pregnant women, or attendance at school and vaccinations for children. The cash transfer is therefore explicitly linked to behaviours that improve health. And with such successes as a more than 50 percent reduction in infant mortality and a 100 percent grade school enrolment, the Bolsa has become a model for reducing extreme poverty across developing countries.

In the world of global development, where the communities in question are often extremely poor, a Basic Income Guarantee in the form of a universal cash transfer makes sense to me. But here in Canada, where the progressive income tax system is well established and most people earn more than the minimum required for a decent standard of living, I favour the guaranteed annual income/negative income tax model. There are attractive aspects of a universal cash transfer, but the upfront cost of a transfer to all Canadians would be very high.

However, despite the cost, we may see a universal cash transfer implemented in other developed countries in the coming years, starting with Finland. In response to changes in the Finnish labour market, the government has called for a universal basic income experiment, which should be launched in 2017. The stated goal of the experiment is to find ways of adapting the social security system so that it provides an incentive to work, while reducing bureaucracy and better organizing their existing multifaceted benefits system. The Dutch city of Utrecht, among others, has also announced its plan to launch a basic income experiment.

Either way, whether negative income tax or universal cash transfer, a Basic Income Guarantee would be a big improvement over our current situation. And it would be very, very good for our health.

———

Basic Income Guarantee pilots have been done all over the world. The signal Canadian example was carried out in Manitoba.

In the 1960s and 1970s, the extent of poverty among seniors and other groups across North America was becoming a significant concern. South of our border, building on the momentum of President Lyndon Johnson's "war on poverty," the Office of Economic Opportunity ran four Basic Income Guarantee experiments; and in Canada, Prime Minister Pierre Trudeau's Liberal government decided to launch its own. The newly elected Ed Schreyer, Manitoba's first ever NDP premier, and his cabinet of young social justice advocates were happy to volunteer their province as the site for the experiment. In 1974 the project was introduced in Winnipeg and in the small farming community of Dauphin. The federal government picked up three-quarters of the cost, and the province the remainder. They called the experiment Mincome.

The purpose of Mincome was to determine the effect of offering a guaranteed income on work effort. Would people quit their jobs? Would the costs of the program balloon as people dropped out of the workforce?

In Winnipeg, a small proportion of the total population was chosen to participate. For comparison, participants were matched to people just like them who continued to use the existing set of social programs.

In Dauphin, they tested a different model: everyone who lived in the town of ten thousand received the same guarantee. A comparator group of people was selected from nearby communities to complete various surveys but did not receive support. In Dauphin, any individual who had no income from any source would receive an income of approximately 60 percent of the Low Income Cut-Off (the unofficial poverty line). As their earned income increased by one dollar, benefits would be reduced by fifty cents until they disappeared entirely. Payouts to the families were indexed to the cost of living and would therefore rise with the inflation rate—a detail that became important as oil prices suddenly rose in the 1970s, leading to high inflation, high interest rates, and high unemployment.

The unanticipated high levels of unemployment meant that more families sought more assistance than anticipated. When Mincome researchers approached the federal and provincial governments for more funding, they found that priorities had changed. Provincially, in 1976, the Schreyer government lost to the Sterling Lyon Conservatives, who weren't interested in helping out a struggling NDP research project. The families continued to receive support, but the research aspect of the project came to an end.

Not long after Mincome ended in Dauphin, scholars from the University of Manitoba dug into the data to examine the work outcomes for Winnipeg participants. Much like their U.S. counterparts who scrutinized results from the American experiments, they found very little reduction in the number of hours people worked in response to having a guaranteed income.

In other words, the fear that the money would impel people to stop working wasn't borne out. Two groups, however, did reduce their hours worked: married women who used the income to "buy" themselves longer maternity leaves (which at the time were in the four- to six-week range) and "young, unattached males" who reduced their work effort substantially and *stayed in school instead*.

Most of the remaining Mincome data sat in boxes in a warehouse for over thirty years.

Enter Dr. Evelyn Forget, a health economist at the University of Manitoba. Professor Forget is a quiet, unassuming person with a Cheshire cat's smile and a mammoth intellect. In 2006, she decided it was time to learn about the impact of Mincome in Dauphin. Using databases only now available in the twenty-first century, she was able to reconstruct the story. In particular, she used data available through Manitoba's universal health care system—which was fully operational by 1971—to understand the impacts on health.

The Forget research team compared the outcomes of people who lived in Dauphin to people with similar characteristics who lived in similar communities in other parts of Manitoba at that time.

The results were striking.

Before Mincome came along, residents of Dauphin were 8.5 percent more likely to be hospitalized than people like them in the neighbouring communities. But by the end of the program, this hospitalization gap had completely disappeared. In other words, having access to a guaranteed annual income reduced the likelihood of ending up in hospital by more than 8 percent. This reduction in health care use was in part due to a decline in accidents and injuries. Mental health visits also declined, both in hospital and in family doctors' offices.

Overall, the reduction reflected a decrease in health care use across the *entire population of Dauphin*—including those who fell below the income cut-off and received the Basic Income Guarantee as well as those who did not.

This is because what makes the Basic Income Guarantee tick isn't simply the money in people's pockets, though that certainly makes a difference in putting food on the table or paying the electricity bill. Income security also means that even those families that never collect a penny know that if they were to fall on hard times they wouldn't lose everything—and this has positive health effects on the whole community. It's known as the "social multiplier effect": if something is good for many of your neighbours, the positive effects spill over to you as well.

If we had discovered a drug, a test, or a surgery that reduced hospitalization rates in Canada by 8.5 percent, we'd be trumpeting it from the rooftops and implementing it nationwide immediately.

The effects extended beyond health services. Before 1974, high school dropout rates were higher in rural Manitoba (including Dauphin) than in Winnipeg. But during Mincome, grade twelve enrolment in Dauphin soared: by 1976 it exceeded 100 percent, as dropouts returned to high school to graduate. After Mincome ended, grade twelve enrolment dropped back down to previous levels, consistent with the rest of rural Manitoba.

On the other side of the world and much more recently, a project was launched in 2008 in Malawi's Zomba District, where the community struggles with high rates of HIV and other sexually transmitted diseases and young women often don't finish school. Researchers recruited unmarried women between the ages of thirteen and twenty-two to participate in a cash transfer program that would provide them (as well as their parents) with monthly financial support. Some received this money in exchange for keeping up a regular attendance in school, while others received it unconditionally. The results were inspiring. The girls in both groups were more likely to enrol in school and to report stronger English-language skills. They were also much less likely to contract HIV or genital herpes infections. By empowering girls financially, their sexual and reproductive health improved, and so did their life chances. These results echo the Mincome findings in that they point to a Basic Income Guarantee as a way to drive up education rates and improve health.

———

The Basic Income Guarantee isn't a pipe dream. In Canada, we already have one for seniors: Old Age Security and the Guaranteed Income Supplement. We also have one for families with children, called the Canada Child Benefit.

As Hugh Segal tells the story, in 1975 in Ontario, we had a poverty rate among seniors of 35 percent, most of whom were women. The Bill Davis government implemented a tax-based seniors' income top-up that then spread across the country and formed the basis of our current Old Age Security program. In three years the poverty rate among seniors dropped from 35 percent to 3 percent. There are very few social policy decisions in our lifetime that have had this kind of impact.

Today, all Canadian seniors essentially receive a basic income: an Old Age Security amount that decreases depending on their income from other sources, and an additional top-up for low-income seniors—the Guaranteed Income Supplement. For 80 percent of seniors aged sixty-five to sixty-nine, these benefits are a primary source of income. They need that money to eat. Food insecurity drops from 23 percent before their sixty-fifth birthdays to 12 percent when they turn sixty-five and start receiving their cheques.

At the other end of the age spectrum, most Canadian families with children receive a monthly cheque from the government through the Canada Child Benefit. The amounts aren't enough for a family to live on, but for the lowest income families it's a substantial supplement—and as you would expect, it improves health. Families that receive the child benefits have better school test scores, mental and maternal health, and other advantages. Interestingly, there are stronger effects on mental health for girls, whereas educational and physical health are more affected for boys.

Taken together, the Canada Child Benefit, Old Age Security, and the Guaranteed Income Supplement essentially offer a Basic Income Guarantee to around one-third of the Canadian population. What is left now is to close the gap so that every Canadian can be protected from the health effects of poverty.

What would it cost? That would depend on where we set the floor. Some have suggested that an appropriate Basic Income Guarantee in the year 2013 would have been somewhere around $20,000 for every Canadian adult and $6000 for every child. If one were to use the 2016

Low Income Cut-Off as a measure of poverty, the amount for a family of four would be just over $45,000.

None of these estimates are intended to be precise, but they can give us a sense of both the number of Canadians who would be eligible and the approximate costs. According to some estimates, the incremental cost to the public purse would be $30 billion to $40 billion annually. Other estimates have ranged from $12 billion to $58 billion. In other words, the cost will depend on how the program is designed—but it will be significant. Regional factors would need to be taken into account, and of course the program would need to be indexed to inflation from the outset, or it wouldn't reduce poverty for long.

On the other hand, by implementing a Basic Income Guarantee we could eliminate a number of existing costly programs—notably social assistance (which includes welfare and some parts of disability support). The relief gained by so many other spending areas that are driven by poverty would also be substantial: the estimated cost of poverty to health care budgets alone in Canada has been assessed at $7.6 billion per year.

By dissolving some programs, recouping some of the savings from other parts of the health and social services systems, saving on administration, and investing some of our collective wealth, we could design a Basic Income Guarantee that would deliver a huge return on investment.

———

One of the concerns often expressed about the Basic Income Guarantee is that it might remove, or diminish, the incentive to work. As we've seen, the Mincome evidence does not bear that out. International research yields the same result: people given a Basic Income Guarantee use it as the springboard for building themselves a better life. In Namibia, with a basic income, self-employment jumped 300 percent. In Liberia, one-third of basic income recipients started their own businesses. In India, those who received a basic income were twice as likely to increase their productive work as those who did not. As columnist

Andrew Coyne has pointed out, "The real disincentive to work arises not from giving money to people who don't work, but taking it away from them when they do." By designing programs that don't claw back benefits by $1 for every $1 earned, the incentive to work is maintained.

Another concern often expressed by detractors of the Basic Income Guarantee is that it would be spent on "inappropriate" items like alcohol, cigarettes, and drugs. Yet in Brazil, families spend the money they get from the Bolsa Família on food, clothes for their children, and school materials. In Kenya, when people living in poverty were given cash unconditionally, 90 percent of them used it to start their own businesses or to purchase livestock.

Would low-income Canadians spend a basic income on beer and popcorn, as one political adviser once put it? Since we already have this program for low-income families with kids, we don't have to wonder. We can look to how people who receive the Canada Child Benefit spend it. This benefit is intended to support low-income kids, but of course it supports low-income families with kids—the money is transferred to low-income parents, who have no restrictions on how they can spend it. Researcher Mark Stabile at the University of Toronto and his colleagues have looked at this question. What they found was that low-income families that receive the benefit spend it like this: on food, on rent, and on transportation. In fact, spending on alcohol and tobacco *declines* when families receive the Canada Child Benefit.

These results are consistent with research showing that alcohol and tobacco consumption may be tied to financial hardship. In fact, after the World Bank looked at all cash transfer studies all over the world, it reported that "almost without exception, studies find either no significant impact or a significant negative impact of (cash) transfers on temptation goods" (such as tobacco and alcohol). One such study—among many others—found that mothers in the U.S. who received a cash supplement smoked less than mothers who didn't. Poverty is stressful. Relieve the poverty, and you reduce the stress and its many ill health effects, including the drive to smoke.

The Basic Income Guarantee idea is catching on across the country—and it's backed by all sides of the political spectrum and at all levels of government. Liberals, Conservatives, New Democrats, and the Greens have all voiced their support for pilots or proposals. Mayors from all over Canada have called for pilot projects, which isn't surprising, since the effects of poverty are often seen in the strain on municipal services, like shelters and food banks.

Now we just have to do it.

How would we design it? Who would receive it? What should the levels be, and how gradually should they phase out? Are there ways to recoup or shift dollars saved from other social programs to help pay for it?

These are all good questions. And given that the Mincome experiment results are now over forty years old, we need pilot projects to help us design such a program for a twenty-first-century Canada. Active discussions are underway about such pilots, in Ontario and elsewhere.

Like medicare, a Basic Income Guarantee is a form of insurance against hard times, a policy that is both simple and fair. The same principles that led us to establish universal health insurance underpin it: administrative simplicity, risk pooling, reliability, dignity for the recipients, and the belief that access to some basic things should be automatic—a right of citizenship rather than an act of charity.

BIG IDEA 6

JONAH: THE ANATOMY OF CHANGE

From Pilot Project to System Solution

Jonah was an "interesting case." That's something nobody wants to be.

He needed a kidney transplant, but the multiple blood transfusions he'd received over the fifty-six years of his life had put him at risk of reacting badly to other people's tissues, making him what we call a "highly sensitized patient." Like hundreds of other Canadians experiencing kidney failure, Jonah's circumstances prevented him from finding a potential match among the limited number of organs available for transplant in his region. The kidney he needed was of a very rare type.

So Jonah had no choice. He continued coming in to the hospital for dialysis three times a week, and waited for a kidney to come up that would be a match for him. This meant going to the dialysis unit at his local hospital, parking the car, spending several hours hooked up to the dialysis machine while he read a book or played cards, and then driving home. He couldn't take on a steady job with that kind of time commitment every week. He was nervous about going on vacation because he didn't want to be too far from his dialysis centre. He felt as if he might never be free to live independently again.

Dialysis is expensive for patients and for the health care system. Every time a kidney is transplanted, allowing a person to come off dialysis, the system saves approximately $70,000 per patient per year. But Jonah relied on dialysis for *fifteen years* because a match was so hard to find.

I heard about Jonah from my colleague Dr. Graham Sher, who is the CEO of Canadian Blood Services. Before CBS began to address the challenge of patients like Jonah, it had to wait for that rare match to come up. Luckily for Jonah, something happened: after so many years of waiting, a suitable kidney from a deceased donor was found through a new approach called the Highly Sensitized Patient program, and Jonah got his transplant.

HSP is a cross-country organ-sharing program developed by Canadian Blood Services in collaboration with provincial transplant programs and health system partners. It has given real hope to highly sensitized patients like Jonah, who now have priority access to a broader national pool of organs for transplant. Without this large-scale approach, these patients would likely continue to live decades of their lives on wait lists, literally tethered to their dialysis machines and with a much shortened life expectancy.

The work of Canadian Blood Services is all about innovation on a large scale. Born out of the tainted blood scandals of the 1970s and 1980s, the organization achieves levels of performance nationally that no single provincial system can achieve on its own. Blood and organ donation programs can't succeed as small, local projects. National programs share scarce resources across geographic boundaries, coordinate access, and ensure safety and consistency.

How does CBS do this? By creating *systems* that overcome parochialism and turf wars. These systems use data to support and improve performance; they use information technology to connect silos rather than just make them more efficient; and they engage providers, especially doctors, in order to standardize their practices and help them take pride in teamwork. That's what efficient systems can do.

For years, Jonah was caught in the nonsystem-ness of medicare. Even though his medical problems were complex, the thing that stood between him and better health wasn't fundamentally medical. It was systemic: regional boundaries and lack of cooperation made it impossible to move from the local to the national scale to find Jonah a kidney. Soon, Canadians who require stem-cell transplantation will be able to benefit from a similar system through the national umbilical cord blood bank.

For Big Ideas to be implemented in health care, we need pan-Canadian systems like the one that helped Jonah. But since much health care delivery resides at the provincial and regional levels and doesn't require large-scale markets to work, we badly need systems at those levels.

In pockets across the country, innovative policy makers, clinical teams, managers, and leaders have done terrific work to improve health care. We've implemented models that work, but—here's the nub of our problem—we've too often done that on a small scale, for a patient with one kind of disease but not another, or in one community but not another.

Examples abound. My own family doctor used to have a six-week wait time just to get in the door for a basic appointment. Two years ago she changed her practice to offer same-day appointments, and I can now consistently get my daughter in to see her on the day I call. (She had to first work down her six-week backlog, and now must make sure she offers enough appointments every week not to develop a backlog again.) Meanwhile, the emergency department at my local pediatric hospital is often filled with kids who couldn't get in to see their own family doctors. In Nova Scotia, a team launched a groundbreaking program that helps frail older people plan for the end of life. But my family friend with dementia who lives in rural Ontario doesn't have access to any such program. In Alberta, a group of hospitals, surgeons, and patients cooperated to reduce wait times for hip and knee replacements. Yet wait times for some other kinds of surgery remain long.

Steven Lewis, a health policy consultant in Saskatoon, keenly observed in an essay he wrote back in 2007 that "the single biggest problem in Canadian healthcare is the failure to apply ingenuity on a grand scale." In other words, we fall down when moving from the project to improve diabetes care, or heart failure, or lung disease in one rural town to the improvement of care for *all* Canadians with that condition. That's what happens when individual parts work well but there isn't a system.

214 BIG IDEA 6

When I asked Steven if he would review and provide feedback on a chapter of this book, he declined pretty emphatically. "There have been lots of sensible books with self-declared big ideas about how to fix the system, and none of them has any influence," he wrote. "The book that needs to be written (if any needs to be written) is a careful, sophisticated political analysis of how change occurs and where there may be opportunities to get done what everyone has said we need to get done."

He had a point. The final Big Idea in this book is actually a precondition of all the others—without it, we can't succeed in any significant reform to medicare. It's time to *build systems that support the implementation of large-scale change.* Most of the time these systems will be at the regional and provincial levels, but in some cases—blood and organ systems, or pharmacare—national systems are needed in order to establish economies of scale and consistency across the country.

———

Elevating a successful innovation beyond the local pilot project or high-performing individual team is what is referred to as "spread and scale."

Spread is the horizontal diffusion of a new way of doing things, either within an organization or more broadly. This is where a new approach catches on as people start to notice how well it's working nearby. We see spread in the fashion world all the time: one day a celebrity is seen wearing her jeans rolled up above her ankle boots, and the next day women all over New York are sporting the same look.

Spread may be an organic process when it concerns ankle boots, but in health care it doesn't simply "happen." It requires a means to disseminate new ideas to other teams that would benefit. It also usually requires local champions, support for teams implementing the idea, and a plan to sustain the changes. The assumption that good ideas can or should be adopted spontaneously has been called the "implementation fallacy." If you want a project to spread beyond the local, you have to be intentional about spreading it.

Scale, on the other hand, is about implementing a single solution across the whole system—often with the stroke of a pen. The Highly Sensitized Patient program that Jonah benefited from is a good example of scale. It requires centralized action by someone who has the power to make the rules. It usually happens across a whole geographic area at once, like a health region or a province or even the country.

In order to improve our health care systems, we need to both spread and scale good ideas.

———

Bernadette is a friend, someone who's known my parents since before I was born. We've always called her our "aunt," even though we're not related by blood. A number of years ago she was admitted to a Canadian hospital for surgery intended to give her a new hip and to even out the length of her legs. One of them was significantly shorter than the other, which had caused the terrible arthritis she now had in both hips. When she woke up from the operation, she did have a new hip—but she discovered that the discrepancy between her leg lengths had doubled. The surgeons had shortened the wrong side.

At first they insisted she was wrong. She was given a protracted explanation about how her muscles had become tight over many years and that it would take a long time for them to relax (I think they were hoping she would relax, too). But eventually the team took responsibility for the error and apologized. She now wears very expensive custom shoes with a platform in one of them to make up for the now three-centimetre difference in her leg lengths.

Wrong-sided surgery happens. This is a critical incident in a hospital, one of those things that everyone agrees should never happen, and it's on the list of personal nightmares for every surgeon and every patient. It ranks up there with injuring an organ or a blood vessel, or causing a patient a significant infection. In a way it's worse, because those things are known complications whereas wrong-sided surgery is a totally avoidable error.

Imagine that in a hospital near you, someone learns that there's a recurring problem: too many people like Bernadette are experiencing avoidable complications of surgery. Maybe a report comes out showing high variations in the frequency of surgical errors, and your local team ranks poorly. Or perhaps a patient like Bernadette goes to the local press.

The surgical team in your hospital calls a meeting, and someone reviews the literature to see what's been shown to work in other settings to make care safer. They decide to implement an approach that has been successful in other places. The team measures the results associated with this change, tracking not just the frequency of surgical errors but also complications like bleeding and infection, rates of death, and patient satisfaction. Over time, they refine the model, and they watch their outcomes improve.

This is how we've ended up with pockets of excellent care across the country. Teams of motivated people come together to redesign care processes because they want to do better. They start with data and a plan, try something different, measure and analyze the impact of those changes, and then continue to modify and improve. They make it a point to sustain the changes. This approach works to improve the quality of patient care.

The surgical safety checklist is a good example of a solution that's been implemented to avoid the kind of error that Bernadette experienced. The concept is simple: the surgical team follows a written checklist to make sure that each and every surgery is done according to plan.

The World Health Organization's surgical safety checklist includes a review at three critical points: before putting the patient to sleep, prior to surgical incision, and again before leaving the operating room. Team members verify—by speaking out loud—a number of key items. They confirm the patient's identity and the surgical procedure to be done (including which side); introduce the members of the surgical team by their name and role; and confirm that medications such as antibiotics have been given when needed. It seems so basic. "This is Bernadette Hayes; she's here today for a hip replacement on the right side; she has no allergies; she's received one gram of Ancef IV [Ancef is an antibiotic sometimes used to reduce the risk of infections that can occur when people have surgery]." Complete the list, and the risk of that person dying decreases by 50 percent—or so the initial studies suggested.

If those large studies were accurate, the next logical step should be to implement surgical safety checklists across the whole health care system, or at least those parts of the system where patients are most likely to benefit. This is where we repeatedly fall down in Canadian health care. Very few health care improvement projects get implemented in a sustainable way, and spread beyond that one area of the organization.

Whose job is it to move a project like the surgical safety checklist beyond the original team? Well, no one in our health care system holds responsibility for this yet. Incentive is lacking: if I can see patients in my office on the same day they call, or my hospital can reduce the number of people who have a bad outcome in surgery, why would I worry about the wait time of the family doctor down the street or the complications in someone else's hospital? This is why the Institute for Healthcare Improvement in the U.S, lists among its "seven spreadly sins" the idea of requiring the person or team who drove the pilot to be responsible for system-wide spread. Teams who made the local change are satisfied, and often lack the skills and the power to be responsible for the spread and scale of the innovation.

For this reason, large-scale change has to be implemented by an organization with teeth, and with a view of the whole system. That can mean the Ministry of Health, the local health authority, the provincial Hospital Association, the College of Physicians and Surgeons, the provincial health quality council, or any number of other organizations.

In July 2010, the Ontario Ministry of Health and Long-Term Care implemented a surgical safety checklist across the entire province. It mandated that hospitals publicly report their use of the checklist. Use of surgical safety checklists then became a national requirement in 2011 for any hospital wanting to receive the stamp of approval from Accreditation Canada, an organization that assesses quality in Canadian health care organizations. In other words, the full power of the scale apparatus was used to implement the tool.

Unfortunately, it didn't work.

At least not in the way it was expected to work. A group of researchers measured whether the implementation of the surgical safety checklist had the desired effect in Ontario. They studied 101 hospitals that performed over a hundred thousand procedures in the three-month period before adoption of a surgical safety checklist and another hundred thousand after its implementation.

None of the hospitals saw a statistically significant reduction in deaths after initiating the use of surgical checklists. There was also no statistical change in post-operative complications. No significant benefit of the use of checklists was found.

The unexpected finding that surgical safety checklists did not make a big difference in Ontario reinforces the importance of rigorously evaluating changes. But of course, beyond knowing that it didn't work, we all wanted to understand *why*.

When a pilot project succeeds in one environment, it's possible that it isn't the innovation itself but rather the special resources put in place to nurture that innovation that make the difference. Maybe when surgical safety checklists were being studied as a research intervention, the fact that teams were participating in research made them pay closer attention to their actions, causing the rate of bad outcomes to decrease.

There's another possibility. As Health Quality Ontario CEO Dr. Joshua Tepper and others have pointed out, the surgical safety checklist was implemented as a classic scale initiative: overnight, every organization was required to do it. The techniques of spread weren't utilized: engaging physicians and teams, building the case for change, rewarding participation, supporting culture change. If the health professionals didn't fully engage, maybe the checklist became just another thing people did by rote. They did it, but they hadn't done the hard work of adapting it to work in their local environments. They didn't "own" the checklist because the scale techniques weren't accompanied by techniques of spread.

————

The surgical safety checklist is a rich example of how complex it can be to move an innovation from the pilot or the research stage to a system-wide solution. Probably nearly every major change in health care requires the use of tools of both spread and scale in order to achieve its full potential. This means we need local champions, local adaptation, local impetus for change, *and* a push and/or support from the centre to ensure that money, rules, incentives, and mandates all point in the same direction.

To get that kind of change—the kind where both spread and scale can happen effectively—we need systems like the ones Canadian Blood Services built for patients like Jonah. High-functioning systems share an anatomy. They have brains: the ability to generate and respond to data. They have hearts: entities with the courage to overcome entrenched interests and to say no when necessary. And they have feet: engaged health care providers who want to participate in change for the better.

Data: The Brain of the System

We collect lots of data in Canadian health care, but we don't do a very good job of sharing it. Most Canadians don't know how their health care experience compares to the "norm." Most doctors don't know how their practice compares to best practice.

Data doesn't change behaviour on its own, but without it we can't know where to focus our attention. When people receive information on how their practice patterns compare to others'—and how they compare to acknowledged "best practices"—something starts to shift inside them.

I have experienced this personally. The first time I participated in an "audit and feedback" project, where I received graphs comparing my performance to others', it was about my patients' access to me. Our clinic had begun measuring the time to the "third next available" appointment, a way to understand how easy it is to see your family doctor in a timely manner. If you call my office to ask for an appointment, the team secretary starts offering you appointment times. Ideally, there should be at least three options available to you in the next couple of days. After you decline the first two options she offers, the third should still be in that twenty-four to forty-eight hour time frame.

I believed that my patients could get in to see me the same week they called. I was dead wrong. It was true that people could be seen quickly by a member of my team if they needed an urgent appointment, but my personal "third next available" time was sixteen days away!

At first, I did what I know a lot of doctors would do: I disputed the data. I was sure that the people collecting the numbers had made a mistake. So when I next went to the clinic, I started asking patients when they'd called to make the appointment we were about to have. Most responded that it had been a couple of weeks. I was shocked.

You may wonder how it's possible that your doctor doesn't know how long you've waited to get an appointment. But I can assure you that in many cases it's highly likely that she has no idea. We show up in clinic, look at the list for that day, and plow through it.

Knowing how long my patients had waited embarrassed me, and it made me want to change my appointment-booking system. That's the magic of audit (monitoring these things) and feedback (showing physicians how they rank in comparison with their peers or best practices). When audit and feedback inspire change, and research shows they often do, it's usually because the feedback includes clear targets and an action plan.

That last point is important. It's no use telling people what's not working well unless you show them how they can fix it. If I'd simply been told that my waiting list was two weeks long without being given any advice on how to reduce it, I'd probably have thrown my hands up and said "I'm working as hard as I can." This isn't just true in family medicine. My specialist colleagues have wait lists that are many months long despite all the hours they put in. Everyone is working hard, so it's difficult not to feel defensive when you're told that your hard work isn't "enough."

Audit and feedback are necessary, but they're not sufficient to make change. We have to give people the tools they need to do their work better. In my case, several members of our team received training from Health Quality Ontario on how to improve same day/next day access for our patients. We spent a few lunch hours learning tips and tricks for matching the supply of appointments to their demand. While those tricks don't solve everything, understanding the factors that commonly

affect waits in a primary practice can help. We figured out that I
needed a few more appointment slots for patients to be seen on
Wednesdays, given that I'm usually not in clinic on Thursdays. When I
go away for a few days to a conference or meeting, a backlog develops,
which means that I need to add extra appointments just before leaving
and on my return. I also looked at the size of my practice to make sure
that the overall number of appointments I was offering in a given
month was sufficient. It was, but the appointments weren't well distributed through the week. I also increasingly use email with my patients,
which keeps appointment slots open for those who really need to be
seen face to face.

When we implemented those changes, I watched my wait time drop
to about half its earlier level, and I'm still trying to bring it down.

Why did it take me so long to recognize the problem and make
changes? The reality is that for many providers and organizations, the
impetus to improve mostly comes from outside their own teams. In my
practice, it was the support from Health Quality Ontario that put us on
the road to improving wait times. We're still slowly learning through the
tools of spread—education and engagement—how to do better. I suspect
that someday those spread techniques will be accompanied by a requirement from the centre—some kind of scale initiative—and perhaps the
pace of change will accelerate. But for the time being, our improvement
work is mostly optional.

The data our team collects about wait times in our practice is confidential. In fact, the doctors on my team don't even know each other's
wait times; when we see the numbers for the team we see them without
any names attached. Taking this approach in the early days, while people
are still getting used to the idea of data collection, can reduce resistance,
but eventually the question arises: when we gather data, to whom should
it be accessible? Local information is intended for quality improvement
purposes and is usually kept fairly confidential, the way employees' eval-
uations go into their HR files and are kept to measure performance but
not shared widely. But data for performance reporting is a different

thing. In an era of transparency and accountability to the people who own our system—citizens—some data ought to be publicly reported.

In Canada this concept is controversial, but internationally it isn't. In the U.S., the Centers for Medicare and Medicaid Services launched its Hospital Compare program more than ten years ago. Hospital Compare publicly reports metrics like hospital infection and readmission rates. A few years later, the Canadian Institute for Health Information launched a much less detailed but more user-friendly website that compares outcomes at the level of health regions or hospitals. Many provincial Ministries of Health have started to post wait times online, sometimes down to the level of the individual surgeon. I recently went on British Columbia's Ministry of Health surgical wait times website to see how long a patient might wait for wrist surgery there, and was able to get the data by surgeon and by hospital.

This is a start, but the websites don't always convey information that matters to patients, who are increasingly interested in hearing the views of other patients who've lived through the same experience. We can expect the internet to generate a fair amount of anecdotal information about people's experiences, but doctor and hospital rating sites aren't exactly scientific. We shouldn't leave all the measurement and reporting up to bloggers and message board discussions.

In trying to communicate information to patients in a meaningful way, some health care groups in the U.S. are now publishing ratings of their physicians on their own websites. For example, the University of Utah Health Care centre emails a twenty-question survey to every single patient who's been treated at one of its clinics within a few days of his or her appointment. They're asked about the friendliness of their provider, the quality of the explanations they were given about their condition and treatment plan, and whether they'd recommend that provider to a friend or family member. Patients can insert their own views in a comment box. Every year UUHC hears back from fifty thousand patients, and it posts all comments, positive or negative, on its website (except those comments that are libelous, slanderous, profane, or risk patient privacy).

In 2015, over 99 percent of all comments received about physicians were posted unedited.

This kind of public reporting takes real courage, and its impact is complex. In the Canadian environment, public reporting, even at the regional level, can lead to all kinds of political trouble. The media and Opposition politicians may jump all over any indication that the system has deficiencies. And at the individual level, every provider worries that one angry patient might unfairly characterize their interaction, or that taking on difficult cases will unfairly skew his or her results. As health reform in the U.S. leads to more and more public reporting of patient experience scores, some doctors have even argued that this can drive them to "do the wrong thing," like caving in to pressure to prescribe unnecessary antibiotics or ordering unnecessary scans in order to bump up patient satisfaction scores.

These are important considerations. But they can't prevent us from moving into a more transparent era. Keeping all the available information confidential is the wrong answer. Surgical complication rates, infection rates, cancer screening rates, immunization rates, patient experience and satisfaction—this information should be available to both patients and providers.

We can begin to get data reporting right by using a broad variety of measures. They must capture the patient experience and be translatable into action and policy changes while also reflecting the complex world in which health care providers and organizations function. And there's a need to account for the complexity of illness correctly, or we risk creating a perverse incentive for doctors to avoid treating the sickest patients.

When we collect the right kinds of data, feed it back to providers and organizations in ways they understand, and publicly report it to support quality improvement, we'll have a functioning brain in the body of medicare. But without the courage to use that information to make change happen, the data won't be enough.

The Heart of the Matter

The heart, as the poetic locus of courage, is a critical component of the anatomy of change.

People are creatures of habit. If I learned as part of my medical training to order a urine test on every patient who comes to my office for a checkup, it would feel unnatural, and somehow less than attentive, for me to stop doing so. I might know that there's no evidence to do it. In fact, it's a waste of money and could harm my patients by picking up meaningless abnormalities that I'd feel compelled to investigate. And yet . . . my hand itches to tick that box on the requisition form. It's also hard for my patients, who might be used to having their urine checked, to feel just as well cared for when I tell them we shouldn't do it anymore.

Yelling louder at doctors to practise "good medicine" or at patients to "use the system responsibly" isn't enough. Decades of research in human psychology and organizational change show that if you want people to change their behaviour, you need to make the *right* thing to do the *easy* thing to do—or perhaps sometimes the *only* thing to do. People need the path of least resistance to be the one that leads to the highest standard of care. They shouldn't be expected to alter their behaviours and their expectations otherwise.

We can't change the way we address the social determinants of health, the organization of primary care, the delivery of services, and their coverage without brave people in governments and health authorities who are willing to help us push for those changes. And in a publicly funded health system nested in a democratic country, governments will muster this courage only when they hear from voters that they should.

The biggest challenge for politicians and governments is saying no to the public. When the evidence shows that stroke units are the best way to deal with acute strokes, that means telling some communities that their local hospital may not offer stroke services anymore because they don't have the full suite of services needed or the volume of patients to warrant it. When the best practice for certain knee injuries points to non-surgical approaches, that means deciding not to pay for the unnecessary operation. People may be upset because their local hospital no longer offers every service, or their neighbour got the procedure five years ago and it was covered then. Deciding to say no, even on the basis of strong evidence and in the interest of reducing variations in care, can quickly lead to a public fight. That's hard, but it doesn't make the decision wrong. These are circumstances where political courage is the only answer.

Hard conversations with voters are just that—hard. But until our politicians are willing to have them and the public is willing to accept that some "local" or "special" solutions can actually hold us back from ensuring the spread and scale of high-quality care, we'll remain in a world where mediocrity looms.

Some jurisdictions create arm's-length agencies to do the heavy lifting. In the U.K., the U.S., and increasingly in Canada, this has been an effective strategy. Allowing regional health authorities, arm's-length agencies like Canadian Blood Services, and Health Quality Councils to make unpopular decisions gives governments some cover. But that means governments have to be willing to cede control and accept those bodies' recommendations even when it's difficult to do so. Citizens have a right to demand that non–democratically accountable organizations do their work based on the best available evidence and free from political and industry interference. We should also applaud political courage when we see it.

Whether it's the Ministry of Health, an arm's-length agency, or a health authority, someone has to be in charge of planning services, identifying problems, and fostering change across the entire system. Without the heart, a system that's designed to support large-scale change can't do its job.

Feet to Do the Walking

In the anatomy of a system for change, clinicians are the feet that do the walking. They can also be the feet that drag.

This is especially, though not exclusively, true of my own profession. Along with nurses, rehab professionals, mental health professionals, and so many others, doctors roll up their sleeves every day to take care of people who need our services, with skill and passion. But unlike many other groups, doctors often see themselves as separate from the system. Until they see themselves as part of it, large-scale change will be blocked.

In an environment where nearly all the money for doctors' payments comes from one source—the government—you'd think Ministries of Health or health regions would somehow be able to require that all patients with a particular condition get access to the same high standard of care.

This is not the case. Canada has a highly decentralized model of health care, with enormous power residing at the level of the individual physician. Ministries of Health, health regions, and hospital CEOs have surprisingly little sway in influencing how doctors practise. The high degree of physician autonomy is the result of our history. In Canada, when doctors were first brought under medicare in Saskatchewan in the 1960s, many resisted the change; a doctors' strike tried to stop the Tommy Douglas government from requiring that they bill the provincial insurance plan for their services rather than having patients use private insurance or pay out of pocket.

In the face of massive public support for medicare, the doctors eventually backed down. But in the compromise that was reached, they wouldn't become employees of the government. Instead, doctors would continue to function as independent entrepreneurs, billing the government for their services but having minimal accountability for the type, number, or quality of those services. Importantly, the money transferred to physicians, unlike the salaries of employees, is purely for the provision of clinical services. There is no requirement to participate in initiatives to improve the quality of care we provide, although in some provinces that's starting to change.

This doesn't mean that doctors can do anything they want without repercussions. Physicians in Canada, like most health professionals, are subject to the policies of our professional colleges. We have to behave ethically, we have to practise medicine within reasonable bounds, and we can't intentionally harm people. Of course, most doctors are skilled professionals who care deeply about their patients and work hard to do right by them. But much of the difference between how two physicians approach the same situation falls into the grey zone of professional preferences, or "practice style." It's unlikely that a physician would be reprimanded for failing to address her long wait time for an appointment using tools that are known to work, or having a Caesarean section rate higher than the norm. It's even less likely when we often don't even know her wait time or her C-section rate.

The result is that physicians have a striking degree of autonomy, even compared to other health care providers. As doctors, we're taught that such autonomy is necessary and desirable. The highly independent nature of medical practice is usually framed within the medical community as a good thing for patient care. The pervasive cultural belief has been that, as independent practitioners, doctors are best able provide patients with the individualized care they need, and that anyone who tries to tell us what to do—administrators, other providers, or the government—is putting some other interest (often financial) ahead of the interests of our patients.

It's laudable to hold tight to the notion that patients' needs come before all else. But physician autonomy has at times been an excuse to either resist important changes that would help patients or passively avoid participating in those changes. The fallacy that patients' needs and the system's needs are mutually exclusive is what's held us back.

Our medical education system has been trying to move with the times, increasing its focus on the profession's social accountability as well as its training in areas like quality improvement. But change takes time. New doctors still graduate into a culture where it's common to view accountability to society for our own practice as optional at best and inappropriate interference at worst.

In training, doctors learn over and over that the individual doctor–patient relationship is a sacred one. I believe this is true. But when it's overemphasized, medical students can come to believe that any outside force is a threat to that critical bond with the patient. It's too easy to interpret this to mean that "the system" is something from which patients must be protected rather than the very infrastructure that allows doctors to care for patients in the first place.

The fact that they function as independent contractors instead of as employees within the system has divided doctors from their colleagues in nursing, allied health, support services, and medical administration. As someone who's chosen to participate in hospital administration, I sometimes see this in the way my own colleagues perceive me. I get angry emails from doctors I've never met who hear me talking about a system issue on the radio and accuse me of having "lost touch" with what it means to be a physician. They assume that because I work for the hospital I can't possibly understand patients' needs, or that because I talk about improving the system I somehow value those needs less than I did when I was solely a clinician.

Because of this mistrust, some doctors—even those who really believe in social accountability—come to see the health care system as something that exists alongside them rather than something of which they're a part. Nurses and doctors are both publicly paid, but in most cases they have very different degrees of accountability: one is an employee of a front-line organization like a hospital or a regional health authority, and the other is paid by a remote entity called "government."

It's time for a new professionalism in medicine, one that is emerging in Canada and needs to be nurtured. It will be built not just on doctors' legitimate devotion to patients, but also on their willingness to participate in improving the system. Dr. Don Berwick has called this professionalism *"an embrace of citizenship in the greater whole that is health care, even when caring for a single patient. . . . This means asking, not just, 'What do I do?' but also, 'What am I part of?'"*

Berwick himself has been lauded as the embodiment of this perspective. An American physician who's held some of the most important leadership roles in that country's health care system, he has that elusive bifocal vision: the ability to see patients up close, in all their vulnerability, and to apply his skills to help them; and the ability to see around him all the broader systemic factors that have led those patients to the moment they're in now.

Indeed, no one has better summarized the duty to see the system beyond the patient than Berwick did in a commencement speech to the 2012 graduating class of Harvard medical school, which he dedicated to his deceased patient, Isaiah:

> Now you don your white coats, and you enter a career of privilege. Society gives you rights and license it gives to no one else, in return for which you promise to put the interests of those for whom you care ahead of your own. That promise and that obligation give you voice in public discourse simply because of the oath you have sworn. Use that voice. If you do not speak, who will?

There are many, many other physicians who feel what Berwick articulates so beautifully—that our role as physicians is not only to take good care of our patients, but also to lead the charge for better social conditions. Many doctors who share that passion don't get involved in such traditional medical politics as sitting on the boards of medical associations, negotiating contracts, and becoming leaders in their hospitals or health teams. Some may instead choose academia and channel their desire for change into their research, or they may participate in important advocacy work outside the mainstream medical community.

We need doctors in all these critical roles, pushing for large-scale system improvement. But we also need doctors who see themselves as citizens to take on traditional medical leadership roles in our hospitals, our primary care teams, and our medical associations. That change is underway, but is by no means complete.

We can nudge progress along, bringing change to medical culture by seeking greater accountability from doctors, paying them differently, and training them in the skills they need to be team players. But the crux of this change has to come from within the medical profession. Our view of our purpose needs to reflect an aspiration not only to heal the patient but to heal the system, as a core aspect of the oath that we swear.

———

Making change is always about the art of the possible. Sometimes it would be great to pass a piece of legislation requiring hospitals or doctors to do something, but it just isn't feasible. At other times it would be better to engage physicians and inspire them to drive change locally, but sometimes they're frankly unwilling or unable to do so. We might have all the goodwill in the world, but the forces aligned against change may be too powerful. Change requires that providers and policy makers be brave when too often we're just tired, trying to get through the day.

The established way of doing things always takes on a life of its own. Organizations and systems develop protocols and procedures that maximize pay or other benefits for the providers or the institution. Change can thus mean a loss of money, power, or prestige for someone, perhaps a doctor, a hospital, or a corporation. The only way to overcome resistance, then, is with a combination of data, political courage, and physician engagement.

Across Canada, health care innovators have proved themselves capable of delivering better care. We know how to do it in our local communities, clinics, and hospitals. The real obstacle in Canadian health care is that we haven't figured out how to do it for everyone, everywhere, all the time.

Unless we can get better at bringing change to every community that needs it, none of the other Big Ideas in this book can be implemented successfully. If we can't effectively spread and scale our success, we can't deliver on the promise of medicare.

Our system generates tons of data, but doesn't yet report it in a timely or public way to stimulate change. So we have only part of a brain. Our policy makers see the need for the spread and scale of successful innovations, but they often lack the courage to make it happen. So we only have part of the heart we need to get the job done. Our physicians are committed to serving patients, but they don't always see it as their job to help improve the system. So our feet can't do the walking.

Implementation of any Big Idea requires us to invest time, energy, and money into that anatomy of change. Each particular Big Idea will also require other body parts to support spread and scale. Information technology, for instance, will often be a necessary connector; well-developed organs are useless without a circulatory system to connect and feed them. Good IT connections can link different environments, making care safer and more efficient. But throwing technology, money, machines, or providers at our problems won't resolve them if the focus always remains local. The building blocks are in place to implement the solutions every Canadian deserves. If the brain, heart, and feet are aligned, things can move.

CONCLUSION

Worthy Action

When my mother arrived in Montreal just before her fourth birthday, her parents faced a tough road ahead. They spoke French and English, but with different accents from those of the locals. They were educated, but they had no credentials or connections that could open doors to stable employment. They were supposed to be looking forward, but when you leave your birthplace, a part of you always looks back. Their plan for a successful and happy life together in Canada went unrealized—not only because of unexpected illness but because of the financial hole it put them in. A high-quality, single-tier, publicly funded health care system wouldn't have eliminated every barrier that stood in the way of my grandfather, Jacques—but it would have helped a lot.

My generation of Canadians doesn't remember what life was like when you had to pay to see a doctor or get hospital care. But our parents and grandparents do. The challenge in those years was to build a system that wouldn't bankrupt a Canadian family with medical bills. We built that through the 1960s, and solidified our commitment to a single-tier system with the passage of the Canada Health Act in 1984. Canadians are—and should be—very proud of that accomplishment.

But more is needed.

When Canadians say, as we consistently do in public polls, that health care is the most important issue for us, we don't just mean that we want more MRI machines or doctors. We want a set of structures that will yield better health for ourselves and our families, so that we can live happy and productive lives. But medicare has become a lightning rod for political conversations that have little to do with health. People who want to see it privatized hide behind claims that our publicly funded model is unsustainable. On the other hand, people who want to see its values preserved can at times be afraid of any kind of change. Medicare is worth fixing, and the fixes are eminently achievable. But for it to be worthy of all the pride we feel in it as a nation, we have work to do.

Almost everyone in this country has strong views about what we should do to improve health care. Some readers will be disappointed that I didn't mention a particular worthy idea they feel passionate about: the need for more mental health services, or the idea of extending public insurance to dental care, or the need to support exercise and healthy eating. Whatever Big Ideas we pursue, they should pass the fundamental test of fulfilling the dual promise of medicare. An improved Triple Aim of better health, better care, and better value grounded in the idea of equity, and solutions worthy of an iconic program.

———

It's a tremendous honour to be a physician in the Canadian health care system, to do work that feels meaningful and to be let into people's lives. Every doctor learns about system issues from her patients. For me, it was patients like Fatou—the pregnant woman using the food bank whom I let down in my residency—and Leslie, my patient with asthma from her substandard housing, who proved to me how factors outside the health care system affect our well-being.

Of course, even if we are able to reduce or eliminate poverty in Canada through a Basic Income Guarantee, people will still get sick. Most disease is identified and managed not in hospitals but where I work: in primary care. Most people still consult their family doctor first. And for people like Abida, my older patient whose complex medical and social needs make her a high user of health care services, a good family doctor can really make a difference. Our tradition of community-based solo family practice has built a foundation, but the twenty-first century demands more of us. The three relationships that form the basis of excellent primary care must be realized: a strong provider–patient relationship, a good connection between the primary care practice and the other parts of the system, and a commitment between the practice and the population it serves.

This means more structure and accountability for the services family doctors provide. I believe that most primary care providers, including doctors, are ready. If we can furnish them with the tools they need to do better and to measure what matters, we'll set them up for success.

As patients (and we're all patients at some point), we must also be willing to participate—which will sometimes mean pushing back. Too often, our conversations about medical interventions focus on their potential benefits without talking about their potential harms. The result is that unnecessary care has become a major source of harm in our health care system—a source of inappropriate intervention, significant side effects, and a waste of time and money. Patients like Sam—the healthy executive who suffered a stroke after an unnecessary angiogram—have paid the price for cavalier ordering of tests and procedures. It's time to change the conversation between health care providers and patients about unnecessary care. Each of us can help by asking good questions about the purpose of tests and treatments and recognizing that more is not always better.

When care *is* necessary to improve health, every Canadian deserves reasonable access to it. That means solutions to wait times that help everyone, not just people who can afford to pay for their care. And it means finally bringing medicines under medicare. Across the country, people like Ahmed the taxi driver are forced to sacrifice their long-term health because of the short-term crunch of prescription drug costs. Alongside that profound inequity lives the uncomfortable truth that we pay some of the highest prices in the world for our prescription medicines. Only our governments can take the necessary steps to establish a national pharmacare program that would ensure access, safety, and appropriate use of medicines at a cost that is affordable not just for governments, but also for citizens and for employers.

For almost any Canadian in our health care system, it's clear that there are aspects that need to be reorganized. With an aging population and the rise of chronic disease on the horizon, we need to reorganize services to keep people out of hospital, out of the emergency department, and better supported in their homes. This should not require more money—we can do much better with the resources we have. We can reduce wait times for specialty care by reorganizing our queues into centralized intake models and including non-doctor providers much more fully in our teams. We can use our emergency departments for emergencies and our hospitals for acutely sick patients, and test new models of care for people whose needs would be better addressed elsewhere. Imagine what more intensive home care would have done for someone like Susan, who cycled in and out of the emergency department and an inpatient hospital bed, finally dying in an ICU connected to lines and tubes. When we creatively reorganize the delivery of care, we'll be able to hit the Triple Aim. When we fail—which we sometimes will—we'll need to learn from those failures rather than denying them.

And when we succeed, every community across Canada should benefit from that success. Governments, regional health authorities, and agencies must scale up successful innovations so that we can reduce the enormous variations in care that exist. Developing *systems* to support spread and scale, rather than just supporting one-off innovative programs, is critical. Where we have created systems to support large-scale change, people like Jonah—whose kidney transplant was finally possible thanks to Canadian Blood Services—have seen very tangible benefits.

Of course, meaningful change has repercussions. The corollary of reducing variation is that we'll need to be prepared to provide people with the care they need but not always all the things they want. Because of this, change will at times require immense political courage. It will also require a new professionalism in medicine, one where doctors are proud to be part of the system, leading change, rather than simply independent practitioners working alongside the system, having change done to them.

The challenges we face—long waits, an aging population, unaffordable drug costs, increasing utilization of services without much improvement in health—can all be solved within a publicly funded health care system. We can stop wasting time on the endless debates about health care zombies like user fees and for-profit care if we focus on the evidence and demonstrate results in the public system. We need to change the channel on the same old debate: less talk about whether medicare is good, more talk about how to make it better.

That can't be the job of government alone. Every Canadian can make choices to improve her or his own health and the health of our kids. We choose health at the individual level by staying active, maintaining a healthy body weight, not smoking, brushing our teeth. We also choose health when we advocate for ourselves and our loved ones in the system by asking questions, participating in our treatment and recovery, and resisting unnecessary care.

Locally, we each choose health when we support programs that ensure that all kids in our local schools get access to a healthy breakfast, lots of activity, and the support they need to complete their education. We choose health at the ballot box by voting for politicians who aren't afraid to be honest about the changes needed in health care—not to privatize it as part of an "adult" conversation, but to improve it as part of being grownups committed to our values. That means making tough choices, as is the case when some providers or corporations have to give up some of their power or profit.

We choose health by demanding that Big Ideas be implemented to improve medicare.

Each of the Big Ideas put forward in this book stands alone; if we were to implement any one of them, we'd see a measurable improvement in the health of Canadians. Taken together, they cover the journey that you and I take through our lives, and are centred in the moments where what we do collectively can have an impact on health.

Even if we do implement all six of these Big Ideas, the health care system in Canada won't be "all better." The work of improving health care is never finished. But I truly believe that these Big Ideas are what we need now to live up to our aspirations. Across the country, dedicated and inspiring people are revamping our medical schools, engaging community members in hospital decision making, reorganizing care to eliminate wait lists, researching best practices, trying new ways of doing things, breaking the old rules to do the very best for patients. We are ready.

No more tinkering around the edges. We know what we need to do. For Canadians like Ahmed, Sam, and Leslie; like Jonah, Susan, and Abida; like you and me, we need to take action worthy of medicare. Let's get started. We have a promise to keep.

ACKNOWLEDGMENTS

Writing this book has been an exercise in humility. People who know much more about each of the issues I raise have been wonderfully generous with their time and advice. My hope is that I've done justice to the patients who inspired each Big Idea and the colleagues and experts who've hoisted me onto their shoulders for a view of the evidence. Anything I've done well here has been because of their help, and I take responsibility for my inevitable missteps.

It takes a village to write a book—or this one, at least. The remarkable physicians and staff of Women's College Hospital deserve credit for their help with the project and for their patience with me as I was writing. This includes the extraordinary team in the Family Practice Health Centre, a group that always pushes to do better for our patients and for each other. My medical and interprofessional colleagues took care of my practice when I wasn't there to do so and have provided me with a wonderful environment in which to grow and learn.

Our CEO, Marilyn Emery, has been a tremendous mentor and supporter of this project—and of me—from the beginning, as has the entire leadership team of the hospital. Kyla Pollack Behar, Melissa Aldham, and Chantale Bielak helped to push the project off the ground and Jennifer Lee, Jacob Ferguson, and Lindsay Reddeman were instrumental in landing it. Lili Shalev Shawn and her team saw that the project was as much a tool for sparking conversation as it was a book, and have put their tremendous skill and passion behind that conversation. Reva Seth also provided extremely valuable advice in that regard, as did Lindsay Mattick and Bob Ramsay. The team at WIHV—the WCH Institute for Health System Solutions and Virtual Care—led by Sacha Bhatia and including Onil Bhattacharyya, Bailey Griffin, Noah Ivers, Jay Shaw, Asad Moten, Hayley Baranek, Ciara Pendrith, and many others, were an inspiration and a resource at many important moments.

I leaned very hard on a group of tremendous experts. Bill Kaplan encouraged me to write the book in the first place, before I thought it could or should be done, and he provided important strategic advice along the way. Many colleagues provided advice, references, or citations in their areas of expertise, including Gary Bloch, Onil Bhattacharya, Irfan Dhalla, Will Falk, Marc-André Gagnon, Joel Lexchin, Laura Pus, and Steven Shrybman. Others talked through tough concepts with me or advised me on structure or strategy: thank you Darrell Bricker, Tony Dean, Terry Fallis, Peter MacLeod, Dave Naylor, and Max Valiquette.

Colleagues provided stories from their own lives or the lives of their patients to illustrate important concepts, including Stacey Daub, Irfan Dhalla, Sarah Giles, Ilana Halperin, Noah Ivers, Carol Kitai, Nick Pimlott, Cara Tannenbaum, Valerie Taylor, Lynn Wilson, my wonderful mother-in-law Lenore Barrett, my brave and brilliant mother, Anita Shilton, and her sister Eliane Shilton. Many kind people did the hard work of editing one or more chapters, including Sacha Bhatia, Adalsteinn (Steini) Brown, Michael Decter, Evelyn Forget, Rick Glazier, Darren Larsen, Michael Law, Wendy Levinson, Steve Morgan, Karen Palmer, Toni Pickard, Nick Pimlott, Hugh Segal, George Southey, Mark Stabile, and Dawn Woodward. A few had the courage to read, and provide comments on, the entire manuscript: Andreas Laupacis, Greg Marchildon, Asad Moten, Joshua Tepper, Karen Palmer, and my gifted and loving father, D'Arcy Martin. Each was generous with time, expertise, encouragement, and honest feedback.

An amazing group of medical trainees—students and residents—assisted with the research for the book. They include Liza Abraham, Manpreet Basuita, Anand Lakhani, Yuchen Li, Vivian Tam, and Henry Zhang. I feel tremendously optimistic that the future of our health care system is in such capable hands.

My friends and colleagues at Canadian Doctors for Medicare also pitched in with edits, assistance, advice, and moral support, especially Karen Palmer and Ryan Meili—who were both amazing as always—but also the executive, board, and staff. CDM is an extended family network across the country that reflects the very best of the medical profession, and it is within that family that I learned how to advocate for health. Of course, advocacy without a rigorous evidence base is of no use—which is why I'm also grateful to the School of Public Policy and Governance at the University of Toronto, where I learned how to rigorously think about and analyze ideas about public policy.

After we first met, I dreamed that my editor, Diane Turbide, helped me bake the perfect cake. My deep gratitude goes to her for understanding me and my message, and making my efforts in the kitchen rise. The tremendous team at Penguin Canada has been a joy to work with. In particular, I'm grateful to freelance copyeditor Karen Alliston, and to Liz Lee, whose skills polished and improved the manuscript. My agent, Chris Bucci, has been an invaluable navigator in this new literary universe, and has become a friend.

To the many patients who inspired this book and continue to teach me how to be a better person and a better doctor, I am extremely grateful.

Living with someone on a mission is never easy. My parents, siblings, extended family, and close friends have been endlessly patient. They brainstormed titles, read passages, gave me space to write, and distracted me when I needed it. Each has peeled me off the ceiling or scraped me off the floor at some point to bring me back to the purpose and to encourage me when I lost my nerve.

But no one can scrape you off the floor like the people you wake up with every morning. For that task, I choose my partner, Steven Barrett, and my daughter, Isa Martin, above all else and every time. For me, they make life better—now and forever.

RECOMMENDED READING

This section is designed for readers who want to delve deeper into any of the Big Ideas. Under each heading I include a short list of my top picks: books, websites, and online articles that I frequently recommend to people who want to learn more, and that are current as of 2016. Some are written for a lay audience, while others are more academic. They don't represent an exhaustive list or cover the whole landscape—they're just my favourites.

THE BASICS

1. For a rigorous overview of the structure, governance, financing and delivery, and quality of Canadian health care, including the Canada Health Act and its implications, see Gregory Marchildon's 2013 book *Health Systems in Transition: Canada*, Second Edition, or Katherine Fierlbeck's 2011 *Health Care in Canada: A Citizen's Guide to Policy and Politics*.

2. For a good snapshot of wait times in Canada, the Wait Time Alliance produces reliable reports, which can be found at www.waittimealliance.ca.

3. Other general dimensions of health system performance can be explored using the interactive tools found on the website of the Canadian Institute for Health Information (CIHI), including the user-friendly site http://yourhealthsystem.cihi.ca.

4. Excellent myth-busters on the aging population, private funding for public wait times, user fees, and other health care zombies can be found in the Canadian Foundation for Healthcare Improvement's Mythbuster series.

BIG IDEA 1   ABIDA: THE RETURN TO RELATIONSHIPS

1. A good way to think about the importance of primary care is to be aware of the "ecology of care": the rates of ill health (chronic conditions) and health

care use among Canadians. Well-known Canadian researcher Moira Stewart and her colleagues have quantified how much we use primary care in relation to other services in their article "Ecology of Health Care in Canada," which was published in *Canadian Family Physician*.

2. A clear and moving articulation of the unique perspective of generalists can be found in a lecture entitled "The Importance of Being Different" by Dr. Ian McWhinney, often thought of as the father of Canadian family medicine. The lecture was published in the *British Journal of General Practice* and is available online.

3. The Four Principles of family medicine (found at www.cfpc.ca/principles) form the basis of the "three relationships for health" and are the foundation of that discipline.

4. A more academic perspective on the same set of issues is set out by Dr. Iona Heath from the U.K. in her lecture "Divided We Fail," which was the 2011 Harveian Oration when she was president of the Royal College of General Practitioners.

5. The seminal works demonstrating that strong primary care systems are associated with better outcomes, fewer disparities, and higher satisfaction in relation to costs were conducted by the late Barbara Starfield and her colleagues. She summarized her work in a paper entitled "Primary Care and Equity in Health: The Importance to Effectiveness and Equity of Responsiveness to People's Needs."

6. More recently and closer to home, Marcus Hollander and colleagues in British Columbia quantified the value of primary care to system costs in their 2009 article "Increasing Value for Money in the Canadian Healthcare System." They found that the sickest patients without a close alignment to primary care incurred an annual system cost of $30,000 each, whereas similar patients with a close alignment to primary care incurred an annual system cost of only $12,000.

7. The changes underway in Canadian primary care are well summarized in an excellent 2011 piece entitled "Primary Health Care in Canada: Systems in Motion" by Brian Hutchison, Jean-Frederic Levesque, Erin Strumpf, and Natalie Coyle (*The Milbank Quarterly,* 89[2], pages 256–288); abstracts of this article can be found online.

8. When it comes to "measuring what matters," the work on the Starfield Model by Dr. George Southey has been adapted and applied by Carol Mulder and other terrific leaders in the Association of Family Health Teams of Ontario. I hope that academic publications on this model will be forthcoming. In the meantime, those who want to learn more about the D2D experiment should start with the pdf entitled "Valuing Comprehensive Primary Care: The Starfield Principles" on the AFTHO website (www.afhto.ca).

9. A good introduction to the concept of population-oriented, relationship-centred primary care can be found in the "Patient's Medical Home" model. The Canadian articulation of this concept (www.cfpc.ca/A_Vision_for_Canada) comes from the College of Family Physicians of Canada.

10. The "Family Medicine for America's Health" initiative commissioned an exhaustive bibliography in order to understand the capacity of primary care to improve America's health care system. The resulting "Primary Care and the Triple Aim" annotated bibliography, produced by the Graham Center, is an extremely thorough look at the evidence relating to primary care and the Triple Aim; it can be found at www.graham-center.org.

BIG IDEA 2   AHMED: A NATION WITH A DRUG PROBLEM

1. The growth of precarious and part-time work in Canada makes the need for pharmacare ever more pressing. In 2015, the Wellesley Institute produced an excellent paper that brings together the important evidence on this topic: "Low Earnings, Unfilled Prescriptions: Employer-Provided Health Benefit Coverage in Canada" can be found at www.wellesleyinstitute.com.

2. For an overview of how over two hundred Canadian academics see the problems of—and the solutions to—prescription medication policy in Canada, I strongly recommend the Pharmacare 2020 report entitled "The Future of Drug Coverage in Canada," which was produced under the leadership of Professor Steve Morgan from the University of British Columbia (and which I had a very small hand in). It can be found at pharmacare2020.ca.

3. For an academic and very thorough analysis of how we've ended up at an impasse on pharmacare and what can be done to get us out of this long-standing rut, I recommend Katherine Boothe's book *Ideas and the Pace of*

Change: National Pharmaceutical Insurance in Canada, Australia, and the United Kingdom.

4. International comparisons of drug prices do not paint Canada in a very favourable light. For a flavour of how big the differential is, see the "Generic Drugs in Canada, 2013" report from the Patented Medicine Prices Review Board. As well, in the Review Board's "Annual Report 2013," see the "Comparison of Canadian Prices to Foreign Prices." Both can be found on the PMPRB website.

5. To learn about the New Zealand experience of bringing prices down for pharmaceuticals, I recommend the highly readable series of background papers listed in "Your Guide to PHARMAC" on the www.pharmac.govt.nz site.

BIG IDEA 3   SAM: DON'T JUST DO SOMETHING, STAND THERE

1. A terrific and highly accessible book for understanding overdiagnosis and the harms of too much medicine is *Overdiagnosed: Making People Sick in the Pursuit of Health* by Dr. H. Gilbert Welch and colleagues.

2. Excellent resources on unnecessary tests and treatments, and how to have a conversation with your doctor about risks and harms, can be found on the Choosing Wisely Canada website (http://choosingwisely.ca); interested readers can also peruse the specialty-specific recommendations on this site.

3. The National Institute for Health and Care Excellence in the U.K. (www.nice.org.uk) also has a well-known "Do Not Do Recommendations" list that covers a variety of areas.

4. For a good academic overview of the problem of overprescribing in the elderly in particular, I recommend the article "Better Prescribing in the Elderly" by Geneviève Lamay and Bill Dalziel at www.canadiangeriatrics.ca.

5. An excellent set of resources on deprescribing can be found at deprescribing.org.

BIG IDEA 4   SUSAN: DOING MORE WITH LESS

1. On methods to redesign health care, including the notion of "pivoting," I recommend Steve Blank's "Why the Lean Startup Changes Everything" from the *Harvard Business Review* (hbr.org) and Brian Golden's "Improving the Patient

Experience Through Design" from the *Rotman Management Journal* (rotman.
utoronto.ca).

2. On the care of high-needs, high-cost individuals, it was Atul Gawande's "The
   Hot Spotters" piece in *The New Yorker* that put this issue on the radar across
   North America, although the skew in health spending was described as early
   as the 1960s in Canada. Gawande's many terrific pieces can be found on *The
   New Yorker* website, and his books are all interesting and eminently readable.

3. A more thorough examination of the issue and some nice infographics can be
   found in the Commonwealth Fund (www.commonwealthfund.org) reports on
   high-needs, high-cost patients, such as the one entitled "Models of Care for
   High-Need, High-Cost Patients: An Evidence Synthesis."

4. In the United States, the Affordable Care Act established the Center for
   Medicare and Medicaid Innovation in order to test innovative payment and
   service delivery models that achieve the Triple Aim for beneficiaries of public
   health care. The stated goal includes a transformation of the American health
   care delivery system "from one that rewards volume of care to one that provides coordinated, patient-centered, and outcome-driven care." An interesting
   perspective on that work so far can be found in Ashish K. Jha's 2015 article
   entitled "Innovating Care for Medicare Beneficiaries: Time for Riskier Bets
   and Embracing Failure."

5. Much has been written about disruptive technology in health care. One of the
   most frequently cited works is Clayton M. Christensen's book *The Innovator's
   Prescription: A Disruptive Solution for Health Care.* His perspective is summarized in an article in the *Harvard Business Review* called "Will Disruptive
   Innovations Cure Health Care?" While I don't subscribe to all his solutions, I
   do find them to be a helpful way to think about which kinds of technology are
   likely to be most useful in redesigning care.

6. On failure in redesigning health care, an entire issue of *HealthcarePapers*
   (www.longwoods.com/publications/healthcarepapers) was released in
   February 2016 on this topic. It was guest co-edited by Dr. Joshua Tepper
   and me.

BIG IDEA 5   LESLIE: BASIC INCOME FOR BASIC HEALTH

1. For an excellent overview of the social determinants of health in Canada, I recommend the book *Social Determinants of Health: The Canadian Facts*, which can be downloaded from www.thecanadianfacts.org.

2. For a seminal work on the Social Determinants of Health, see Michael Marmot and colleagues' "Closing the Gap in a Generation," which can be found on the website of the WHO. Marmot's recent book, *The Health Gap: The Challenge of an Unequal World*, offers a deeply moving account of how the social determinants lead to domestic and global health inequities.

3. Dr. Ryan Meili's book, *A Healthy Society: How a Focus on Health Can Revive Canadian Democracy*, illustrates the importance of the social determinants of health in a highly accessible way. The organization he founded, Upstream, has an excellent website (www.thinkupstream.net) that includes videos, articles, and analysis on current issues relating to the social determinants of health in Canada.

4. The Mincome experiment in Manitoba has been summarized by Professor Evelyn Forget in her paper "The Town with No Poverty."

5. For a comprehensive look at Basic Income literature from an academic perspective, a recommended resource is *Basic Income: An Anthology of Contemporary Research*, edited by Karl Widerquist, Jose A. Noguera, Yannick Vanderborght, and Jurgen De Wispelaere.

6. To learn more about the links between inequality and social problems, the seminal work is Richard G. Wilkinson and Kate Pickett's book *The Spirit Level: Why More Equal Societies Always Do Better*.

7. For more on the effects of poverty on children, see the 2015 article entitled "Association of Child Poverty, Brain Development, and Academic Achievement" by Nicole Hair, Jamie Hanson, Barbara Wolfe, and Seth Pollak.

8. For more on social assistance and its limits, see "Poverty, Health, and Social Assistance" by Andrew Pinto, Gary Bloch, Ritika Goel, and Fran Scott; this 2011 report was a submission to the Committee for the Review of Social Assistance in Ontario.

BIG IDEA 6   JONAH: THE ANATOMY OF CHANGE

1. Variations in health care around the world are a focus of much academic work. A 2014 OECD report entitled "Geographic Variations in Health Care: What Do We Know and What Can Be Done to Improve Health System Performance?" looks at this issue from an international perspective, with Chapter 4 focusing on such variations in Canada.

2. In their 2008 book, *High Performing Healthcare Systems: Delivering Quality by Design*, Ross Baker and colleagues explore a series of case studies of systems that achieve excellence and show the capacity to improve. It is available at longwoods.com.

3. Steven Lewis's essay "Spare the Policy, Spoil the Profession," also hosted at longwoods.com, offers a damning summary of critiques of the way in which health care policy has dealt with the medical profession in Canada.

4. Dennis Kendel is a Canadian doctor who's been very thoughtful about the tension between physician accountability and autonomy; see, for example, his 2014 essay entitled "Are We Afraid to Use Regulatory and Policy Levers More Aggressively to Optimize Patient Safety?"

5. Dr. Atul Gawande from the U.S. has written extensively on this issue. One of my favourites is "Cowboys and Pit Crews," his 2011 commencement speech to the graduating Harvard medical school class. It was published on *The New Yorker*'s website.

6. In his piece "Era 3 for Medicine and Health Care," published in JAMA in 2016, Don Berwick beautifully encapsulates the transition that is upon us in the way we think about our work as doctors and our relationship to the health care system.

CITATIONS

PROLOGUE

2   ***DeBakey had pioneered an experimental procedure*** U.S. Department of
Veterans Affairs. (2015). Michael E. DeBakey VA Medical Center, Houston, Texas.
www.houston.va.gov/debakey.asp

THE BASICS

9   ***Subcommittee on Primary Health and Aging*** U.S. Senate Subcommittee on
Health, Education, Labour, and Pensions. (2016). Subcommittee on Primary Health
and Retirement Security. www.help.senate.gov/about/subcommittees/primary-
health-and-retirement-security

11   ***My remarks ended just shy of the five-minute mark*** National Cable Satellite
Corporation (C-SPAN). (2014). C-Span – International Health Care Models. www.
c-span.org/video/?c4486943/cspan-international-health-care-models

12   ***exchange between Republican Senator Richard Burr and me*** U.S. Senate
Committee on Health, Education, Labor and Pensions. (2014). Subcommittee
hearing. Access and cost: What the US health care system can learn from other
countries. Transcribed from original testimony. www.help.senate.gov/hearings/
access-and-cost-what-the-us-health-care-system-can-learn-from-other-countries

12   ***The Los Angeles Times picked it up under the headline*** Hiltzik, M. (2014).
Watch an expert teach a smug U.S. senator about Canadian healthcare. articles.
latimes.com/2014/mar/12/business/la-fi-mh-watch-a-canadian-20140312

12   ***net influx of physicians from the United States*** Canadian Health Services
Research Foundation. (2008). Myth: Canadian doctors are leaving for the United
States in droves. www.cfhi-fcass.ca/Migrated/PDF/myth29_e.pdf?

12   ***in those areas of Australia where private insurance*** Duckett, S. J. (2005).
Private care and public waiting. *Australian Health Review*, 29(1), 87–93. www.ncbi.
nlm.nih.gov/pubmed/15683360

13   ***I know that there are forty-five thousand in America*** Wilper, A. P.,
Woolhandler, S., Lasser, K. E., McCormick. D., Bor, D. H., & Himmelstein, D. U.

(2009). Health insurance and mortality in US adults. *American Journal of Public Health*, 99(12), 2289–2295. http://www.ncbi.nlm.nih.gov/pmc/articles/PMC2775760/

13   **national hero** Chai, C. (2014, March 13). Doctor who schooled U.S. senator 'thrilled' by Canadian support. *Global News*. globalnews.ca/news/1205831/doctor-who-schooled-u-s-senator-thrilled-by-canadian-support

13   **"Joan of Arc"** Skyvington, S. (2014, May 5). Medicare's Joan of Arc. *The Kingston-Whig Standard*. www.thewhig.com/2014/05/05/medicares-joan-of-arc

14   **a 2012 Leger Marketing poll** Jedwab, J. (2012). Pride in Canadian symbols and institutions. Leger Marketing poll commissioned by the Association for Canadian Studies. https://acs-aec.ca/pdf/polls/Pride%20in%20Canadian%20Symbols%20and%20Institutions.ppt

14   **We can't, the argument goes** Simpson, J. (2012). *Chronic Condition: Why Canada's Health Care System Needs to Be Dragged into the 21st Century*. Toronto: Penguin Group.

15   **"adult discussion"** Mulroney, B. (2010, October, 18). Brian Mulroney—Wanted: Regulatory Czar. *The National Post*. business.financialpost.com/fp-comment/wanted-regulatory-czar

15   **"Building on Values"** Commission on the Future of Health Care in Canada. (2002). Building on Values: The Future of Health Care in Canada – Final Report. publications.gc.ca/collections/Collection/CP32-85-2002E.pdf

16   **If you understand who's paying** Evans, R. (1998). Going for gold: The redistributive agenda behind market-based health care reform. *The Nuffield Trust*. www.nuffieldtrust.org.uk/sites/files/nuffield/publication/Going_for_Gold.pdf

16   **About 70 percent of Canadian health care** Canadian Institute for Health Information. (2005). National Health Expenditure Trends, 1975 to 2015. www.cihi.ca/sites/default/files/document/nhex_trends_narrative_report_2015_en.pdf

17   **every province has established a single-payer insurance scheme** Parliament of Canada. (2005). The Canada Health Act: Overview and Options. www.lop.parl.gc.ca/content/lop/researchpublications/944-e.htm

17   **A small but not insignificant number of people are not eligible** Goel, Ritika, Bloch, Gar & Paul Caulford. (2013). Waiting for care. Effects of Ontario's 3-month waiting period for OHIP on handed immigrants. *Canadian Family Physician*, 59(6). & Caulford, P., & D'Andrade, J. (2012). Health care for Canada's medically uninsured immigrants and refugees: Whose problem is it? *Canadian Family Physician*, 58(7), 725–727.

17–18   **principles of the Canada Health Act** Canada Health Act (1985, c. C-6). (2012). Department of Justice Canada. laws-lois.justice.gc.ca/PDF/C-6.pdf

19   **an estimated 18 percent of the premiums** Jiwani, A., Himmelstein, D., Woolhandler, S., & Kahn, J. G. (2014). Billing and insurance-related administrative costs in United States' health care: Synthesis of micro-costing evidence. *BMC Health Services Research*, 14(556). www.biomedcentral.com/1472-6963/14/556

19   **Administrative costs are a lot higher** Woolhandler, S., Campbell, T., & Himmelstein, D. U. (2003). Costs of health care administration in the United States and Canada. *New England Journal of Medicine* 349, 768–75. www.nejm.org/doi/full/10.1056/NEJMsa022033#t=article

20   **hospital-based physicians like me are under much more direct control from the state** Cribb, J., Emmerson, C., & Sibieta, L. (2014). Public sector pay in the UK. Institute for Fiscal Studies. www.ifs.org.uk/bns/bn145.pdf

21   **in recent years more for-profit primary care** Mehra, N. (2008). Eroding public medicare: Lessons and consequences of for-profit health care across Canada. www.ontariohealthcoalition.ca/wp-content/uploads/Eroding-Public-Medicare.pdf

21   **this isn't a large, investor-owned business** Deber, R. B. (2002). *Delivering health care services: Public, not-for-profit, or private? Commission on the Future of Health Care in Canada, Background Paper No. 17.* http://publications.gc.ca/collections/Collection/CP32-79-17-2002E.pdf

21   **Canada having a "government monopoly"** Fayerman, P. (2015, February 10). Dr. Brian Day #1: Everything you need to know about him and his legal case against the government health care "monopoly." *The Vancouver Sun.* http://blogs.vancouversun.com/2015/02/10/dr-brian-day-1-everything-you-need-to-know-about-him-and-his-legal-case-against-the-government-health-care-monopoly

22   **women have more difficulty accessing some services** Pelletier, R., Humphries, K. H., Shimony, A., Bacon, S. L., Lavoie, K. L., Rabi, D., Karp, I., Tsadok, M. A., & Pilote, L. (2014). Sex-related differences in access to care among patients with premature acute coronary syndrome. *Canadian Medical Association Journal, 186*(7), 497–504. http://www.cmaj.ca/content/early/2014/03/17/cmaj.131450

22   **People in rural communities, those living in poverty** National Collaborating Centre for Aboriginal Health. (2011). Access to Health Services As A Social Determinant of First Nations, Inuit, and Métis Health. www.nccah-ccnsa.ca/docs/fact%20sheets/social%20determinates/Access%20to%20Health%20Services_Eng%202010.pdf & Ontario Council of Agencies Serving Immigrants. (2005). Canada's Health Care Debate – The Impact on Newcomers. http://w.ocasi.org/downloads/OCASI_health_care_policy_position.pdf & Ontario Ministry of Health and Long-Term Care. (2011). Rural and Northern Health Care Report Executive Summary. www.health.gov.on.ca/en/public/programs/ruralnorthern/docs/exec_summary_rural_northern_EN.pdf

23   **Our provinces and territories have primary responsibility** Health Canada. (2012). Canada's Health Care System. www.hc-sc.gc.ca/hcs-sss/pubs/system-regime/2011-hcs-sss/index-eng.php

24   **In order to receive federal funding for health care, provinces have to adhere** Canada Health Act (1985, c. C-6). (2012). Department of Justice Canada. laws-lois.justice.gc.ca/PDF/C-6.pdf

24   **agreements called Health Accords** Government of Canada. (2006). First minis-
      ters' meeting on the future of health care 2004: A 10-year plan to strengthen health
      care. http://healthycanadians.gc.ca/health-system-systeme-sante/cards-cartes/
      collaboration/2004-meeting-racontre-eng.php

24   **For on-reserve First Nations and Inuit communities** Report of the Auditor
      General of Canada. (2015). Report 4—Access to Health Services for Remote First
      Nations Communities. www.oag-bvg.gc.ca/internet/English/parl_oag_201504_04_
      e_40350.html

25   **This can create divided systems of care** Marchildon, G. P., Katapally, T. R.,
      Beck, C. A., Abonyi, S., Episkenew, J., Pahwa, P., & Dosman, J. A. (2015). Exploring
      policy driven systemic inequities leading to differential access to care among
      Indigenous populations with obstructive sleep apnea in Canada. *International Journal
      for Equity in Health, 14,* 148. www.ncbi.nlm.nih.gov/pmc/articles/PMC4683910

25   **Indigenous peoples in Canada continue to have much worse health out-
      comes** Health Canada. (2016). First Nations and Inuit Health. Diseases and condi-
      tions. www.hc-sc.gc.ca/fniah-spnia/diseases-maladies/index-eng.php & King, M.,
      Smith, A., & Gracey, M. (2012). Indigenous health part 2: The underlying causes of
      the health gap. *The Lancet, 374,* 76–85. http://cahr.uvic.ca/nearbc/documents/2009/
      lancet-vol374-2.pdf

25   **doctors are not allowed to "extra bill"** Marchildon, G. P. (2014). The three
      dimensions of universal Medicare in Canada. *Canadian Public Administration, 57*(3),
      362–382. onlinelibrary.wiley.com/doi/10.1111/capa.12083/abstract;jsessionid=D4955
      C63362498F4201A874B29FBCA4B.f03t04?userIsAuthenticated=false&deniedAccess
      CustomisedMessage=

26   **It's set in negotiations between the government and the medical association**
      Government of Ontario. (2016). Health Insurance Act, R.R.O. 1990, Reg. 552:
      General. www.ontario.ca/laws/regulation/900552

26   **A 2015 report from the Organisation for Economic Co-operation and
      Development** Organisation for Economic Co-operation and Development. (2015).
      Health at a glance 2015. Remuneration of doctors, ratio to average wage, 2013. www.
      keepeek.com/Digital-Asset-Management/oecd/social-issues-migration-health/
      health-at-a-glance-2015_health_glance-2015-en#page91

26   **a "brain drain" of doctors south of the border** Canadian Institute for Health
      Information. (2014). Physicians in Canada, 2013: Summary report. https://secure.
      cihi.ca/free_products/Physicians_In_Canada_Summary_Report_2013_en.pdf

28   **The term Triple Aim** Berwick, D. M., Nolan, T. W., & Wittington, J. (2008). The
      Triple Aim: Care, health, and cost. *Health Affairs, 27*(3), 759–769. http://content.
      healthaffairs.org/content/27/3/759.full

29   **Indigenous peoples and some other marginalized groups** National
      Collaboration Centre for Aboriginal Health. (2013). Setting the Context: An

Overview of Aboriginal Health in Canada. www.nccah-ccnsa.ca/Publications/Lists/
Publications/Attachments/101/abororiginal_health_web.pdf

29   *The proportion of Canadians who say they are in good or excellent health*
Health Council of Canada. (2014). Where you live matters: Canadian views on
health care quality. www.healthcouncilcanada.ca/content_lm.php?mnu=2&mnu1=4
8&mnu2=30&mnu3=56

29   *Our average life expectancy is just over eighty-one years* Organisation for
Economic Co-operation and Development. (2015). Health at a glance 2015. www.
oecd.org/health/health-systems/health-at-a-glance-19991312.htm

29   *Canada comes in sixth place* Nolte, E., & McKee, M. C. (2008). Measuring the
health of nations: Updating an earlier analysis. *Health Affairs*, 27(1), 58–71. http://
content.healthaffairs.org/content/27/1/58.full

29   *When compared to thirty-four OECD countries* Organisation for Economic
Co-operation and Development. (2015). Health at a glance 2015. www.keepeek.com/
Digital-Asset-Management/oecd/social-issues-migration-health/health-at-a-glance-
2015_health_glance-2015-en#page55

30   *Over the last ten years we've done much better* Canada Health Infoway.
(2015). The path of progress. Annual report 2014–2015. www.infoway-inforoute.ca/en/
component/edocman/resources/i-infoway-i-corporate/annual-reports/2771-annual-
report-2014-2015

31   *fewer than half of Canadians* Health Council of Canada. (2014). Where you live
matters: Canadian views on health care quality. www.healthcouncilcanada.ca/
content_lm.php?mnu=2&mnu1=48&mnu2=30&mnu3=56

31   *The methods used to compare health care in different countries* Docteur,
E., Berenson, R. A. (2009). How Does the Quality of U.S. Health Care Compare
Internationally? Timely Analysis of Immediate Health Issues. www.urban.org/sites/
default/files/alfresco/publication-pdfs/411947-How-Does-the-Quality-of-U-S-Health-
Care-Compare-Internationally-.PDF

31   *According to the annual Wait Time Alliance report cards* Wait Time
Alliance. (2015). WTA Reports. www.waittimealliance.ca/wta-reports

32   *Some countries with two-tier systems have long waits* Flood, C. M. (2001).
Profiles of Six Health Care Systems: Canada, Australia, The Netherlands, New
Zealand, The UK, and The US. http://www.parl.gc.ca/Content/SEN/Committee/371/
soci/rep/volume3ver1-e.pdf.

32   *In 2013 (the latest year for which data are available at the time of writing)*
Canadian Institute for Health Information. (2015). National Health Expenditure
Trends, 1975 to 2015. www.cihi.ca/sites/default/files/document/nhex_trends_
narrative_report_2015_en.pdf

33   *For every dollar we spend on health care in Canada* Canadian Institute
for Health Information. (2015). National Health Expenditure Trends, 1975 to 2015.

www.cihi.ca/sites/default/files/document/nhex_trends_narrative_report_2015_
en.pdf

33   **U.K., where eighty-three cents** Organisation for Economic Co-operation and
Development. (2013). OECD.Stat: Health Status. http://stats.oecd.org/index.
aspx?DataSetCode=HEALTH_STAT

33   **United States, which has the highest private spending** Canadian Institute for
Health Information. (2015). National Health Expenditure Trends, 1975 to 2015. www.
cihi.ca/sites/default/files/document/nhex_trends_narrative_report_2015_en.pdf

33   **We have very low levels of public funding** Organisation for Economic
Co-operation and Development. (2015). Health at a glance 2015. www.keepeek.com/
Digital-Asset-Management/oecd/social-issues-migration-health/health-at-a-
glance-2015_health_glance-2015-en#page36 & Quiñonez, C. (2013). Why was dental
care excluded from Canadian Medicare? *Network for Canadian Oral Health Research
Working Papers Series, 1*(1).

33   **Since 1998, our average out-of-pocket health care expenses** Sanmartin, C.,
Hennessy, D., Lu, Y., & Law, M. R. (2014). Trends in out-of-pocket health care
expenditures in Canada, by household income, 1997 to 2009. *Statistics Canada*.
www.statcan.gc.ca/pub/82-003-x/2014004/article/11924-eng.pdf

33   **has been called the Pac-Man argument** Drummond, D. & Burleton, D. (2010).
Charting a path to sustainable health care in Ontario. 10 proposals to restrain cost
growth without compromising quality of care. *TD Economics*. www.td.com/
document/PDF/economics/special/td-economics-special-db0510-health-care.pdf

33   **"straight lines of death" fallacy** Falk, W., Mendelsohn, M., Hjartarsen, J. &
Stoutley, A. (2011). Fiscal Sustainability and the Transformation of Canada's
Healthcare System: A Shifting Gears Report. *The Mowat Centre*. mowatcentre.ca/
fiscal-sustainability-canadas-healthcare/

34   **Our total spending on health care is now falling** Canadian Institute for
Health Information. (2015). National health expenditures trends, 1975 to 2015.
www.cihi.ca/sites/default/files/document/nhex_trends_narrative_report_2015_en.pdf

34   **This made the fraction** Evans, R. (1998). Going for gold: The redistributive agenda
behind market-based health care reform. *The Nuffield Trust*. www.nuffieldtrust.org.
uk/sites/files/nuffield/publication/Going_for_Gold.pdf

35   **And these days, as citizens have pushed for better** Navigator. (2016).
Navigator poll shows widespread support for infrastructure spending. www.navltd.
com/insights/navigator-poll-shows-widespread-support-infrastructure-spending/

35   **we can expect to see health care costs grow by about 1 percent per year**
Mackenzie, H., & Rachlis, M. (2010). The sustainability of medicare. *Canadian
Federation of Nurses Unions*. https://nursesunions.ca/sites/default/files/Sustainability.
web_.e.pdf

35   **The biggest increase in health care costs** Canadian Institute for Health

Information. (2015). National health expenditure trends, 1975 to 2015. www.cihi.ca/
sites/default/files/document/nhex_trends_narrative_report_2015_en.pdf

35   **Every Canadian adult, of every age group** Health Council of Canada. (2009).
Value for money: Making Canadian health care stronger. www.healthcouncilcanada.
ca/tree/2.49-HCC_VFMReport_WEB.pdf

36   **On average, each year we spend about C$6000 per person** Canadian
Institute for Health Information. (2015). National Health Expenditure Trends,
1975 to 2015. https://secure.cihi.ca/free_products/nhex_trends_narrative_
report_2015_en.pdf

37   **we're one of the top ten spenders** Organisation for Economic Co-operation and
Development. (2015). Health at a glance 2015. www.keepeek.com/Digital-Asset-
Management/oecd/social-issues-migration-health/health-at-a-glance-2015_health_
glance-2015-en#page166

39   **Morris Barer and Bob Evans first coined the term** Barer, M., Evans, R. G.,
Hertzman, C., & Johri, M. (1998). Lies, damned lies and health care zombies:
Discredited ideas that will not die. HPI Discussion Paper #10, University of Texas,
Houston Health Science Center.

39   **these fees deter both unnecessary and necessary care** Keeler, E. B., & Rolph,
J. E. (1983). How cost sharing reduced medical spending of participants in the health
insurance experiment. *Journal of the American Medical Association*, 249(16), 2220–2222.
www.rand.org/pubs/external_publications/EP19830401.html

39–40 **One U.S. study looked at how employees** Brot-Goldberg, Z. C., Chandra, A.,
Handel, B. R., & Kolstad, J. T. (2015). What does a deductible do? The impact of
cost-sharing on health care prices, quantities, and spending dynamics. The National
Bureau of Economic Research Working Paper No. 21632. http://eml.berkeley.edu/
~bhandel/wp/Utilization_BCHK_Web.pdf

40   **In the late 1960s the Saskatchewan government** Beck, R. G. & Horne, J. M.
(1980). Utilization of publicly insured health services in Saskatchewan, during and
after copayment. *Medical Care*, 18(8), 787–806. www.jstor.org/stable/3764080?seq=1#
page_scan_tab_contents

40   **a drop most marked among people who could least afford to pay** Beck, R. G.,
& Horne, J. M. (1980). Utilization of publicly insured health services in Saskatchewan
before, during and after copayment. *Medical Care*, 18(8), 787–806. www.jstor.org/
stable/3764080?seq=1#page_scan_tab_contents

40   **user fees reduce usage of the kind of health care** Creese, A. (1997). User fees:
They don't reduce costs, and they increase inequity. *British Medical Journal*, 315(7102),
202–203. www.ncbi.nlm.nih.gov/pmc/articles/PMC2127164/pdf/9253259.pdf

41   **fail to produce significant revenues** Stabile, M., & N-Marandi, S. (2010). Fatal
flaws: Assessing Quebec's failed health deductible proposal. *C.D. Howe Institute*.
www.cdhowe.org/pdf/Working_Paper_Stabile.pdf

41   ***once you start setting fees*** Birch, S. (2004). Charging the patient to save the
       system? Like bailing water with a sieve. *Canadian Medical Association Journal,*
       170(12), 1812–1813. www.ncbi.nlm.nih.gov/pmc/articles/PMC419770/

41   ***A study was conducted in Australia*** Duckett, S. J. (2005). Private care and
       public waiting. *Australian Health Review, 29*(1), 87–93. www.ncbi.nlm.nih.gov/
       pubmed/15683360

41   ***when Manitoba experimented briefly*** DeCoster, C., MacWilliam, L., & Walld, R.
       (2000). Waiting times for surgery: 1997/98 and 1998/99 update. *Manitoba Centre for*
       Health Policy and Evaluation. mchp-appserv.cpe.umanitoba.ca/reference/waits2.pdf

42   ***private health insurance does not improve access*** Canadian Medical
       Association Task Force on the Public–Private Interface. (2006). It's about access:
       Informing the debate on public and private health care. www.cwhn.ca/en/node/
       27868#sthash.kPDer2x9.dpuf

43   ***the number of private clinics inside the public system is growing*** Mehra, N.
       (2008). Eroding Public Medicare: Lessons and Consequences of For-Profit Health
       Care Across Canada. http://www.ontariohealthcoalition.ca/wp-content/uploads/
       Eroding-Public-Medicare.pdf

43   ***In the United States, being admitted*** Devereaux, P. J., Choi, P. T. L., Lacchetti,
       C., Weaver, B., Schünemann, H. J., Haines, T., Lavis, J. N., Grant, B. J. B., Haslam,
       D. R. S., Bhandari, M., Sullivan, T., Cook, D. J., Walter, S. D., Meade, M., Khan,
       H., Bhatnagar, N., & Guyatt, G. H. (2002). A systematic review and meta-analysis of
       studies comparing mortality rates of private for-profit and private not-for-profit hospi-
       tals. *Canadian Medical Association Journal, 166*(11), 1399–1406. www.cmaj.ca/
       content/166/11/1399.full

43   ***dialysis in a for-profit*** Devereaux, P. J., Schünemann, H. J., Ravindran, N.,
       Bhandari, M., Garg, A. X., Choi, P. T. L., Brydon, J. B. G., Haines, T., Lacchetti, C.,
       Weaver, B., Lavis, J. N., Cook. D. J., Haslam, D. R. S., Sullivan, T., & Guyatt, G. H.
       (2002). Comparison of mortality between private for-profit and private not-for-profit
       hemodialysis centers: A systematic review and meta-analysis. *Journal of the*
       American Medical Association, 288(19), 2449–2457. http://jama.jamanetwork.com/
       article.aspx?articleid=195538

43   ***a 2015 study looked at the rates of hospitalization and death*** Tanuseputro,
       P., Chalifoux, M., Bennett, C., Gruneir, A., Bronskill, S. E., Walker, P., & Manuel,
       D. (2015). Hospitalization and mortality rates in long-term care facilities: Does for-
       profit status matter? *Journal of the American Medical Directors Association, 16*(10),
       874–883. Epub 2015 Sep 30. www.jamda.com/article/S1525-8610(15)00414-4/abstract

45   ***Most European nations invest more public money*** Organisation for Economic
       Co-operation and Development. (2015). Health at a glance, 2015. www.keepeek.com/
       Digital-Asset-Management/oecd/social-issues-migration-health/health-at-a-glance-
       2015_health_glance-2015-en#page167

45   **In France, having private insurance** Chevreul, K., Durand-Zaleski, I., Bahrami,
      S., Hernández-Quevedo, C., & Mladovsky, P. (2010). France: Health System Review.
      Health Systems in Transition, 12(6). www.euro.who.int/__data/assets/pdf_file/0008/
      135809/E94856.pdf

45   **In Germany, only 10 percent of the population** Greß, S. (2007). Private health
      insurance in Germany: Consequences of a dual system. *Health Policy, 3*(2), 29–37.
      www.ncbi.nlm.nih.gov/pmc/articles/PMC2645182

45   **earn more money than doctors in many European countries** Organisation
      for Economic Co-operation and Development. (2015). Health at a glance 2015. www.
      keepeek.com/Digital-Asset-Management/oecd/social-issues-migration-health/
      health-at-a-glance-2015_health_glance-2015-en#page91

45   **clauses that preserve the ability of Canadian governments** Government
      of Canada. (1994). North American Free Trade Agreement. www.international.
      gc.ca/trade-agreements-accords-commerciaux/agr-acc/nafta-alena/index.aspx?
      lang=eng

BIG IDEA 1

54   **"In hospitals, the diseases stay"** Heath, I. (2006, January). Keeping the particular
      alive in general practice. *Irish College of General Practitioners.* www.icgp.ie/assets/26/
      D2AF6FE9-DEFF-4524-9ABEADC5FB3B7AC4_document/Iona.pdf

55   **For many kinds of care** Yeravdekar, R., Yeravdekar, V. R., & Tutakne, M. A.
      (2012). Family physicians: Importance and relevance. *Journal of the Indian Medical
      Association, 110*(7), 490–493. europepmc.org/abstract/med/23520678

56   **"A death from a non-cardiac cause"** Health, I. (2011). Divided we fail. *Clinical
      Medicine, 11*(6), 576–86. www.clinmed.rcpjournal.org/content/11/6/576.full

56   **Systems that focus on good primary care** Martin, D., Pollack, K., & Woolard,
      R. F. (2014). What would an Ian McWhinney health care system look like? *Canadian
      Family Physician, 60*(1), 17–19. www.cfp.ca/content/60/1/17.full.pdf

56   **people are living longer** Heath, I., & Sweeney, K. (2005). Medical generalists:
      Connecting the map and the territory. *British Medical Journal, 331*(7530), 1462–1464.
      www.ncbi.nlm.nih.gov/pubmed/16356984

56   **one study that looked at men . . . with severe, uncontrolled high blood
      pressure** Shea, S., Misra, D., Ehrlich, M. H., Field, L., & Francis, C. K. (1992).
      Predisposing factors for severe, uncontrolled hypertension in an inner-city minority
      population. *New England Journal of Medicine, 327,* 776–781. www.nejm.org/doi/
      full/10.1056/NEJM199209103271107#t=article

56   **Study after study has confirmed** Starfield, B., Shi, L., & Macinko, J. (2005).
      Contribution of primary care to health systems and health. *Milbank Quarterly, 83*(3),
      457–502. www.ncbi.nlm.nih.gov/pmc/articles/PMC2690145/

56   ***A man was referred to me*** Barron, L. (2015, February 28). Why you need a family
      doctor. By a surgeon. canadianfemalesurgeon.wordpress.com/2015/02/28/why-you-
      need-a-family-doctor-by-a-surgeon

57–58 ***More than two hundred Canadian adults out of every thousand*** Stewart,
      M., & Ryan, B. (2015). Ecology of health care in Canada. *Canadian Family Physician,*
      61(5), 449–453. www.cfp.ca/content/61/5/449.full

58   ***High-performing health care systems*** Baker, G. R., & Denis, J. (2011,
      September). A comparative study of three transformative healthcare systems:
      Lessons for Canada. CHSRF Commissioned report. www.cfhi-fcass.ca/sf-docs/
      default-source/commissioned-research-reports/Baker-Denis-EN.pdf?sfvrsn=0

58   ***approximately 85 percent of Canadians report*** Canadian Institute for Health
      Information. (2012). Health Care in Canada 2012 A: Focus on Wait Times. www.cihi.
      ca/en/hcic_2012_pptx_en.pptx

58   ***nearly three-quarters of those surveyed in 2013*** Health Council of Canada. (2013).
      Where you live matters: Canadian views on health care quality. Results from the 2013
      Commonwealth Fund International Health Policy Survey of the General Public. www.
      healthcouncilcanada.ca/content_lm.php?mnu=2&mnu1=48&mnu2=30&mnu3=56

59   ***their training enables them*** Huftless, S., & Kalloo, A. N. (2013). Screening colo-
      noscopy: A new frontier for nurse practitioners. *Clinical Gastroenterology and
      Hepatology, 11*(2), 106–108. www.ncbi.nlm.nih.gov/pubmed/23142205 & Mundinger,
      M. O., Kane, R. L., Lenz, E. R., Totten, A. M., Tsai, W. Y., Cleary, P. D., Friedewald,
      W. T., Siu, A. L., & Shelanski, M. L. (2000). Primary care outcomes in patients
      treated by nurse practitioners or physicians: A randomized trial. *Journal of the
      American Medical Association, 283*(1), 59–68. http://www.ncbi.nlm.nih.gov/
      pubmed/10632281 & Ministry of Health and Long Term Care. (2016). Health work-
      force planning and regulatory affairs division. Mid career. New roles in nursing.
      www.health.gov.on.ca/en/pro/programs/hhrsd/nursing/mid_career.aspx

60   ***in Canada in the early 1990s*** Joschko, J., & Busing, N. (2016). Exploring the fac-
      tors that influence the ratio of generalists to other specialists in Canada. *Canadian
      Family Physician, 62*(3), E122–128. www.cfp.ca/content/62/3/e122.abstract

61   ***"a robust appreciation . . ."*** Heath, I., & Sweeney, K. (2005). Medical generalists:
      Connecting the map and the territory. *British Medical Journal, 331*(7530), 1462–1464.
      www.ncbi.nlm.nih.gov/pubmed/16356984

61   ***"a perception of something being wrong . . ."*** Heath, I. (2010). World
      Organization of Family Doctors (Wonca) perspective on person-centered medicine.
      International Journal of Integrated Care. www.globalfamilydoctor.com/GetFile.aspx?
      oid=FBC397FA-3287-4E6D-9F82-E0CEE179AD6F

61   ***Primary care providers like family doctors see more illness than disease***
      Heath, I., & Sweeney, K. (2005). Medical generalists: Connecting the map and the
      territory. *British Medical Journal, 331*(7530), 1462–1464.

62   **the patient–physician relationship is central** The College of Family Physicians of Canada. (2015). Four principles of family medicine. www.cfpc.ca/ProjectAssets/Templates/Category.aspx?id=885&langType=4105&terms=Family+medicine+is+a+community-based+discipline

62   ***"the relationship is usually prior . . ."*** McWhinney, I. R. (1996). The importance of being different. William Pickles Lecture. *British Journal of General Practice, 46*(408), 433–436. www.ncbi.nlm.nih.gov/pmc/articles/PMC1239699/

63   ***health care systems centred on primary care*** Starfield, B., Shi, L., & Macinko, J. (2005). Contribution of primary care to health systems and health. *Milbank Quarterly, 83*(3), 457–502. www.ncbi.nlm.nih.gov/pmc/articles/PMC2690145/

65   ***the real value and importance of the primary care relationship*** Devoe, J. E., Nordin, T., Kelly, K., Duane, M., Lesko, S., Saccocio, S. C., & Lesser, L. I. (2011). Having and being a personal physician: Vision of the Pisacano Scholars. *Journal of the American Board of Family Medicine, 24*(4), 463–468. www.ncbi.nlm.nih.gov/pmc/articles/PMC3211082/

66   ***something that happens when the door clicks shut*** Berwick, D. M. (2012). To Isaiah. *Journal of the American Medical Association, 307*(24), 2597–2599. http://jama.jamanetwork.com/article.aspx?articleid=1199158

67   ***such as screening for and treating high blood pressure*** McAlister, F. A., Wilkins, K., Joffres, M., Leenen, F. H. H., Fodor, G., Gee, M., Tremblay, M. S., Walker, R., Johansen, H., & Campbell, N. (2011). Changes in the rates of awareness, treatment and control of hypertension in Canada over the past two decades. *Canadian Medical Association Journal, 183*(9), 1007–1013. www.ncbi.nlm.nih.gov/pmc/articles/PMC3114892/

67   ***Specialists are three times more likely*** Allan, G. M., Kraut, R., Crawshay, A., Korownyk, C., Vandermeer, B., & Kolber, M. R. (2015). Contributors to primary care guidelines: What are their professions and how many of them have conflicts of interest? *Canadian Family Physician, 61*(1), 52–58. http://www.cfp.ca/content/61/1/52.full

67   ***recommended preventive services*** Yarnall, K. S. H., Pollak, K. I., Østbye, T., Krause, K. M., & Michener, J. L. (2003). Primary care: Is there enough time for prevention? *American Journal of Public Health, 93*(4), 635–641. www.ncbi.nlm.nih.gov/pmc/articles/PMC1447803/

67   ***recommended manoeuvres*** Østbye, T., Yarnall, K. S., Krause, K. M., Pollak, K. I., Gradison, M., & Michener, J. L. (2005). Is there time for management of patients with chronic diseases in primary care? *Annals of Family Medicine, 3*(3), 209–214. www.ncbi.nlm.nih.gov/pubmed/15928223

67   ***family doctor could spend between eleven and eighteen hours*** Pimlott, N. (2008). Who has time for family medicine? *Canadian Family Physician, 54*(1), 14–16. www.cfp.ca/content/54/1/14.full

73   *RACE—Rapid Access to Consultative Expertise* What is RACE?
      www.raceconnect.ca/what-is-race

74   *about three-quarters of primary care doctors* Canadian Institute for Healthcare
      Information. (2015). How Canada Compares: Results from the Commonwealth Fund
      2015 International Health Policy Survey of Primary Care Physicians. www.cihi.ca/
      sites/default/files/document/2015-cmwf-chartpackenrev-web.pptx

76   *primary care needs to incorporate elements* Price, D., Baker, E., Golden, B.,
      & Hannam, R. (2015, May). Patient Care Groups: A new model of population based
      primary health for Ontario. *A report on behalf of the Primary Health Care Expert
      Advisory Committee.* www.oma.org/Resources/Documents/primary_care_price_
      report.pdf

78   *Ontario project called D2D* Association of Family Health Teams of Ontario
      (AFHTO). (2015). D2D 2.0 report release: AFHTO members advance primary care
      measurement. www.afhto.ca/highlights/key-issues/d2d-2-0-report-release/

79   *He called this the "Starfield observation"* Southey, G. (2013). A Path to
      Greater Effectiveness, Efficiency and Equity In Ontario's Health Care System
      Through Stable Primary Care Relationships, Provider Accountability And Measured
      Outcomes: Economic Perspectives of Controlling Health Costs and Assuring
      Quality. www.dorvalmedical.ca/wp-content/uploads/2012/01/Economic-Perspectives-
      of-Controlling-Health-Costs-2013-04-18.pdf

81   *only about a third of family doctors* The College of Family Physicians of Canada,
      Canadian Medical Association, & The Royal College of Physicians and Surgeons
      of Canada. (2013). National Physician Survey, 2013. Results for Family Physicians.
      http://nationalphysiciansurvey.ca/wp-content/uploads/2013/09/2013-FPGP-EN-Q6a.pdf

81   *Ontario's auditor general found* Office of the Auditor General of Ontario.
      (2011). Ministry of Health and Long-Term Care. Chapter 3, Section 3.06. Funding
      Alternatives for Family Physicians. www.auditor.on.ca/en/content/annualreports/
      arreports/en11/306en11.pdf

81   *jeopardize patient access and make waits for primary care longer*
      Baerlocher, M. O., Noble, J., & Detsky, A. S. (2007). Impact of physician income
      source on productivity. *Clinical and Investigative Medicine, 30*(1), 42–43. http://
      cimonline.ca/index.php/cim/article/view/448/564

82   *Every option encourages some behaviours* Peckham, S., & Gousia, K. (2014).
      GP payment schemes review. *PRUComm, a collaboration between London School of
      Hygiene and Tropical Medicine, the University of Manchester, and the Centre for
      Health Services Studies, University of Kent.* www.kent.ac.uk/chss/docs/GP-payment-
      schemes-review-Final.pdf

82   *over 40 percent of medical degrees were earned* The Association of Faculties
      of Medicine of Canada. (2014). Canadian medical education statistics, 2014. www.
      afmc.ca/pdf/CMES2014-Complete-Optimized.pdf

82   *we see fewer patients per day* Cohen, M., Ferrier, B. M., Woodward, C. A., & Goldsmith, C. H. (1991). Gender differences in practice patterns of Ontario family physicians (McMaster medical graduates). *Journal of the American Medical Women's Association, 46*(2), 49–54. http://www.ncbi.nlm.nih.gov/pubmed/2033207 & Roter, D. L., Hall, J. A., & Aoki, Y. (2002). Physician gender effects in medical communication: A meta-analytic review. *Journal of the American Medical Association,* 288(6), 756–764. http://jama.jamanetwork.com/article.aspx?articleid=195191

82   *During our reproductive years* Barer, M. L., Evans, R. G., & Hedden, L. (2014). False hope for Canadians who study medicine abroad. Canadian Medical Association Journal, 186(7), 552. www.cmaj.ca/content/186/7/552

83   *new physicians have little interest* The College of Family Physicians of Canada, Canadian Medical Association, & The Royal College of Physicians and Surgeons of Canada. (2012). The 2012 National Physician Survey for Medical Residents. http://nationalphysiciansurvey.ca/wp-content/uploads/2013/02/NPS2012-Resident-Full-EN.pdf

83   *only 1 percent of new family medicine graduates* The College of Family Physicians of Canada, Canadian Medical Association, & The Royal College of Physicians and Surgeons of Canada. (2012). The 2012 National Physician Survey for Medical Residents. http://nationalphysiciansurvey.ca/wp-content/uploads/2013/02/NPS2012-Resident-Full-EN.pdf

BIG IDEA 2

90   *Canada is the only developed country* Morgan, S. G., Daw, J. R., & Law, M. R. (2013). Rethinking pharmacare in Canada. www.cdhowe.org/pdf/Commentary_384.pdf

91   *overmedication and inappropriate prescribing* Morgan, S. G., Hunt, J., Rioux, J., Proulx, J., Weymann, D., & Tannenbaum, C. (2016). Frequency and cost of potentially inappropriate prescribing for older adults: a cross-sectional study. *Canadian Medical Association Journal Open,* 4(2), E346.

91   *mostly an accident of history* Boothe, K. (2015). *Ideas and the Pace of Change: National Pharmaceutical Insurance in Canada, Australia, and the United Kingdom.* Toronto: University of Toronto Press. www.utppublishing.com/Ideas-and-the-Pace-of-Change-National-Pharmaceutical-Insurance-in-Canada-Australia-and-the-United-Kingdom.html

91   *one-third of Canadian adults live with at least one chronic condition* Health Council of Canada. (2007). A Health Outcomes Report. Why Health Care Renewal Matters: Learning from Canadians with Chronic Health Conditions. www.healthcouncilcanada.ca/tree/2.20-Outcomes2FINAL.pdf

91   *HIV medications for people who are HIV positive* Detels, R., Muñoz, A., McFarlane, G., Kingsley, L. A., Margolick, J. B., Giorgi, J., Schrager, L. K., & Phair, J. P. (1998). Effectiveness of potent antiretroviral therapy on time to AIDS and death

in men with known HIV infection duration. *Journal of the American Medical Association,* 280(17), 1497–1503. & Johnston, K. M., Levy, A. R., Lima, V. D., Hogg, R. S., Tyndall, M. W., Gustafson, P., Briggs, A., & Montaner, J. S. (2010). Expanding access to HAART: A cost-effective approach for treating and preventing HIV. *AIDS,* 24(12), 1929–1935. www.ncbi.nlm.nih.gov/pubmed/20588171

91   **inhalers for people with asthma** Rebuck, A. S. (2013). The global decline in asthma death rates: Can we relax now? *Asia Pacific Allergy Journal,* 3(3), 200–203. www.ncbi.nlm.nih.gov/pmc/articles/PMC3736367

91   **cardiac medicines for people who've had a heart attack** Flather, M. D., Yusuf, S., Kober, L., Pfeffer, M., Hall, A., Murray, G., Torp-Pedersen, C., Ball, S., Pogue, J., Moyé, L., & Braunwald, E. (2000). Long-term ACE-inhibitor therapy in patients with heart failure or left-ventricular dysfunction: A systematic overview of data from individual patients for the ACE-Inhibitor Myocardial Infarction Collaborative Group. *The Lancet,* 355(9215), 1575–1581. www.ncbi.nlm.nih.gov/pubmed/10821360 & Furberg, C. D., & Pitt, B. (2001). Are all angiotensin-converting enzyme inhibitors interchangeable? *Journal of the American College of Cardiology,* 37(5), 1456–1460. http://content.onlinejacc.org/article.aspx?articleid=1127138 & Taylor, F., Huffman, M. D., Macedo, A. F., Moore, T. H., Burke, M., Davey Smith, G., Ward, K., & Ebrahim, S. (2013). Statins for the primary prevention of cardiovascular disease. *Cochrane Database of Systematic Reviews, 1.* www.ncbi.nlm.nih.gov/pubmed/23440795

92   **Low-income people with diabetes** Booth, G. L., Bishara, P., Lipscombe, L. L., Shah, B. R., Feig, D. S., Bhattacharyya, O., & Bierman, A. S. (2012). Universal drug coverage and socioeconomic disparities in major diabetes outcomes. *Diabetes Care,* 35(11), 2257–2264. www.ncbi.nlm.nih.gov/pmc/articles/PMC3476904

92   **the more people have to spend on their prescriptions** Goldman, D. P., Joyce G. F., & Zheng, Y. (2007). Prescription drug cost—associations with medication and medical utilization and spending and health. *Journal of the American Medical Association,* 298(1), 61–69. http://jama.jamanetwork.com/article.aspx?articleid=207805

93   **drug coverage becomes a factor in people's career and job choices** McGroarty, G. (2011). Benefits versus salary: Which is worth more? *Sun Life Financial.* www.sunlife.ca/ca/Learn+and+Plan/Money/Financial+planning+tips/Benefits+versus+salary+Which+is+worth+more?vgnLocale=en_CA

93   **it's called "job lock"** Frakt, A. (2014). Job lock: Introduction. http://theincidentaleconomist.com/wordpress/job-lock-introduction

94   **Nearly three-quarters of part-time workers** Barnes, S. & Anderson, L. (2015). Low earnings, unfilled prescriptions: Employer-provided health benefit coverage in Canada. *The Wellesley Institute.* www.wellesleyinstitute.com/wp-content/uploads/2015/07/Low-Earnings-Unfilled-Prescriptions-2015.pdf

94   **Young people and women, who are more likely** Ferrao, V. (2010, December). "Paid work," in Women in Canada: A gender-based statistical report. *Statistics Canada*. www.statcan.gc.ca/pub/89-503-x/2010001/article/11387-eng.pdf & Statistics Canada. (2015). Part-time employment rates, chart G.2. www.statcan.gc.ca/pub/71-222-x/2008001/sectiong/g-part-partiel-eng.htm

94   **most Canadians with jobs are excluded** Barnes, S., & Anderson, L. (2015). Low earnings, unfilled prescriptions: Employer-provided health benefit coverage in Canada. *The Wellesley Institute*. www.wellesleyinstitute.com/wp-content/uploads/2015/07/Low-Earnings-Unfilled-Prescriptions-2015.pdf

95   **a patient with congestive heart failure** Demers, V., Melo, M., Jackevicius, C., Cox, J., Kalavrouziotis, D., Rinfret, S., Humphries, K. H., Johansen, H., Tu, J. V., & Pilote, L. (2008). Comparison of provincial prescription drug plans and the impact on patients' annual drug expenditures. *Canadian Medical Association Journal, 178*(4), 405–409. www.cmaj.ca/content/178/4/405.full

95   **one in five Canadian households** Angus Reid Institute. (2015). Prescription drug access and affordability an issue for nearly a quarter of all Canadian households. http://angusreid.org/prescription-drugs-canada

95   **two-thirds of Canadians over the age of sixty-five** Canadian Institute for Health Information. (2014). Drug use among seniors on public drug programs in Canada, 2012. https://secure.cihi.ca/free_products/Drug_Use_in_Seniors_on_Public_Drug_Programs_EN_web_Oct.pdf

95   **22 percent of our prescription drug costs** Canadian Institute for Health Information. (2014). Drug spending in 2014. www.cihi.ca/web/resource/en/nhex_2014_infosheet_en.pdf

95–96 **one in ten Canadians does not fill a prescription** Law, M. R., Cheng, L., Dhalla, I. A., Heard, D., & Morgan, S. G. (2012). The effect of cost on adherence to prescription medications in Canada. *Canadian Medical Association Journal, 184*(3), 297–302. http://www.cmaj.ca/content/early/2012/01/16/cmaj.111270

96   **3 percent of the Dutch and 2 percent of the British** Gagnon, M-A. (2014). *A roadmap to a rational pharmacare policy in Canada*. Ottawa: Canadian Federation of Nurses Unions. https://nursesunions.ca/sites/default/files/pharmacare_report.pdf & Schiff, G. D. (2013). A piece of my mind. Crossing boundaries—violation or obligation? *Journal of the American Medical Association, 310*(12), 1233-1234. www.ncbi.nlm.nih.gov/pubmed/24065007

98   **new classes of on-patent drugs** Morgan, S. G., Bassett, K. L., Wright, J. M., Evans, R. G., Barer, M. L., Caetano, P. A., & Black, C. D. (2005). "Breakthrough" drugs and growth in expenditure on prescription drugs in Canada. *British Medical Journal, 331*, 815–816. www.bmj.com/content/331/7520/815

101   **goes for about $800 in Canada** Ontario Ministry of Health and Long-Term Care. (2016). Ontario Drug Benefit Formulary/Comparative Drug Index. Retrieved

April 2015 from www.formulary.health.gov.on.ca/formulary/results.xhtml?q=Lipitor
&type=2

101   *A year's supply of the exact same drug* New Zealand Pharmaceutical Management
Agency (PHARMAC). (2016). Online Pharmaceutical Schedule. Retrieved April 2015
from www.pharmac.govt.nz/Schedule?osq=Atorvastatin&code=C0732041137

101   *Canadians pay 30 percent more* Patented Medicine Prices Review Board. (2013).
Annual Report 2013, Comparison of Canadian Price to Foreign Prices. http://www.
pmprb-cepmb.gc.ca/view.asp?ccid=938#1765

101   *Drug prices in Canada are among the highest* Beall, R. F., Nickerson, J. W., &
Attaran, A. (2014). Pan-Canadian overpricing of medicines: A 6-country study of cost
control for generic medicines. *Open Medicine* 8(4). www.openmedicine.ca/article/
view/645/566

103   *Some policy makers have argued that maintaining high patented drug
prices encourages* Government of Canada. (2015). Patented Medicine Prices
Review Board: Strategic plan 2015–2017. www.pmprb-cepmb.gc.ca/view.asp?ccid=1197

103   *The more we've spent on pharmaceutical products* Government of Canada.
(2014). Patented Medicine Prices Review Board. Annual report 2014. www.pmprb-
cepmb.gc.ca/view.asp?ccid=1217#a8 & Lexchin, J. (2003). Intellectual property rights
and the Canadian pharmaceutical marketplace: Where do we go from here? www.
policyalternatives.ca/sites/default/files/uploads/publications/National_Office_Pubs/
ipr.pdf

103   *Compare this to the U.K., where drug prices are* Kiriyama, N. (2011). Trade and
Innovation: Pharmaceuticals. *Organisation for Economic Co-operation and Development.* www.oecd-ilibrary.org/docserver/download/5kgdscrcv7jg.pdf?expires=14427734
36&id=id&accname=guest&checksum=12893DDCD318DF887B518C2F5A409AE3

104   *Another growing factor in pricing* Sinclair, S., Trew, S., & Mertins-Kirkwood,
H. (2014). Making sense of the CETA: An analysis of the final text of the Canada-
European Union Comprehensive Economic and Trade Agreement. *Canadian Centre
for Policy Alternatives.* www.policyalternatives.ca/publications/reports/making-
sense-ceta

104   *generic drugs . . . are nearly double the median prices* Government of
Canada. (2014). Patented Medicine Prices Review Board. Generic drugs in Canada,
2013. www.pmprb-cepmb.gc.ca/view.asp?ccid=1122

104   *amlodipine is 86 percent lower in New Zealand* Beall, R. F., Nickerson, J. W.,
& Attaran, A. (2014). Pan-Canadian overpricing of medicines: A 6-country study of
cost control for generic medicines. *Open Medicine,* 8(4), E130–E135. www.
openmedicine.ca/article/view/645/566

104   *it's now the norm for governments to pay 18 percent* The Pan-Canadian
Pharmaceutical Alliance. (2016). Background: Generic drugs. www.
pmprovincesterritoires.ca/en/initiatives/358-pan-canadian-pharmaceutical-alliance

105 ***especially where they competitively tender to procure*** Law, M. R., & Kratzer, J. (2013, September 17). The road to competitive generic drug prices in Canada. *Canadian Medical Association Journal, 185*(13), 1141–1144. www.cmaj.ca/content/185/13/1141

105 ***the number of pharmacies in Canada continues to go up*** Labrie, Y. (2015). The Other Health Care System: Four areas where the private sector answers patients' needs. Chapter 2- Pharmacies in Canada: Accessible private health care services. *Montreal Economic Institute.* www.iedm.org/files/cahier0115_en.pdf

106 ***$383 million more per year for generic medications*** Gagnon, M-A., & Hébert, G. (2010, September 13). *The Economic Case for Universal Pharmacare: Costs and Benefits of Publicly Funded Drug Coverage for All Canadians.* Ottawa: Canadian Centre for Policy Alternatives. https://s3.amazonaws.com/policyalternatives.ca/sites/default/files/uploads/publications/National%20Office/2010/09/Universal_Pharmacare.pdf

106 ***$6.8 billion more in premiums*** Law, M. R., Kratzer, J., & Dhalla, I. A. (2014). The increasing inefficiency of private health insurance in Canada. *Canadian Medical Association Journal, 186*(12), E470-474. www.cmaj.ca/content/early/2014/03/24/cmaj.130913.full.pdf+html

106 ***administrative costs . . . 8 percent in the private sector*** Gagnon, M-A. (2014). *A roadmap to a rational pharmacare policy in Canada.* Ottawa: Canadian Federation of Nurses Unions. https://nursesunions.ca/sites/default/files/pharmacare_report.pdf

106 ***General Motors CEO Richard Wagoner*** French, R. (2006, October 29). GM, nation losing out to health care. *The Salt Lake Tribune.* http://archive.sltrib.com/story.php?ref=/healthscience/ci_4567855

106 ***Warren Buffett has looked at the numbers too*** French, R. (2006, October 29). GM, nation losing out to health care. *The Salt Lake Tribune.* http://archive.sltrib.com/story.php?ref=/healthscience/ci_4567855

106 ***GM and Ford paid $1500 per vehicle in health costs*** Daschle, T., Greenberger, S. S., & Lambrew, J. M. (2008). *Critical: What We Can Do About the Health-Care Crisis.* New York: St. Martin's Griffin. https://books.google.ca/books/about/Critical.html?id=MlweIW_sU3EC&redir_esc=y&hl=en

107 ***the insurance industry's association has called for*** Hope, W. (2015). The better way—public and private sectors working together to reform pharmacare in Canada. News release. www.clhia.ca/domino/html/clhia/clhia_lp4w_lnd_webstation.nsf/page/AA2597E98A11A70085257E140047580C

107 ***We've seen exactly this in Quebec*** Gouvernement du Québec. (2015). Eligibility. www.ramq.gouv.qc.ca/en/citizens/prescription-drug-insurance/Pages/eligibility.aspx

107 ***The result has been staggeringly expensive*** Morgan, S. G., Daw, J. R., & Law, M. R. (2013). Rethinking pharmacare in Canada. *C.D. Howe Institute.* www.cdhowe.org/pdf/Commentary_384.pdf

107   **Instead of cost containment, the Quebec approach has resulted in cost-shifting** Gagnon, M-A. (2014). *A roadmap to a rational pharmacare policy in Canada.* Ottawa: Canadian Federation of Nurses Unions. nursesunions.ca/report-study/roadmap-rational-pharmacare-policy-in-canada & Smolina, K., & Morgan, S. (2014). The drivers of overspending on prescription drugs in Quebec. *Healthcare Policy 10*(2), 19-26. www.longwoods.com/content/24046

107   **and there is less bargaining capacity** Gagnon, M-A. (2015, June 26). Quebec should not be the model for national pharmacare. *The Globe and Mail.* www.theglobeandmail.com/opinion/quebec-should-not-be-the-model-for-national-pharmacare/article25135678/

107   **even private insurance companies are struggling** Nelson, J. (2015, July 31). The high-stakes battle of medications, insurers and the government. *The Globe and Mail.* www.theglobeandmail.com/report-on-business/the-high-stakes-battle-of-medications-governments-and-insurers/article25807404

107   **increase in the number of plans adding annual or lifetime maximums** Kratzer, J., Mcgrail, K., Strumpf, E., & Law, M. R. (2013). Cost-control mechanisms in Canadian private drug plans. *Healthcare Policy, 9*(1), 35–43. www.ncbi.nlm.nih.gov/pubmed/23968672

107   **can't afford drug coverage for their employees** Mercer. (2011). Cost trends in health benefits for Ontario businesses: Analysis for discussion. Commissioned by the Ontario Chamber of Commerce for release at the Ontario Economic Summit. www.occ.ca/Publications/Cost-Trends-in-Health-Benefits-Report.pdf

108   **$8.2 billion annually** Morgan, S. G., Law, M., Daw, J. R., Abraham, L., & Martin, D. (2015, March 16). Estimated cost of universal public coverage of prescription drugs in Canada. *Canadian Medical Association Journal 187*(7). www.cmaj.ca/content/early/2015/03/16/cmaj.141564

108   **In 1994, those federal and provincial tax subsidies** Smythe, J. G. (2001, August 19). Tax subsidization of employer-provided health care insurance in Canada: Incidence analysis. Working Paper, Department of Economics, University of Alberta, Edmonton.

109   **Up to 90 percent of new drugs** Light, D. W., & Lexchin, J. R. (2012). Pharmaceutical and research development: What do we get from all that money? *British Medical Journal, 345,* E4348. www.bmj.com/content/345/bmj.e4348

109   **Often called "me too" drugs** Morgan, S. G., Bassett, K. L., Wright, J. M., Evans, R. G., Barer, M. L., Caetano, P. A., & Black, C. D. (2005). "Breakthrough" drugs and growth in expenditure on prescription drugs in Canada. *British Medical Journal, 331,* 815–816. www.bmj.com/content/331/7520/815

109   **the cure rate is up to 96 percent** U.S. Food and Drug Administration. (2014). Approval of Sovaldi (sofosbuvir) tablets for the treatment of chronic hepatitis C. www.fda.gov/ForPatients/Illness/HepatitisBC/ucm377920.htm

109   **the price in Canada of a twelve-week course of therapy** Hepatitis C Education & Prevention Society. (2014). New Canadian Developments Re: Sofosbuvir's price and approval schedule. http://hepcbc.ca/2014/02/updates-canadian-sofosbuvir-pricing-cadth-queuing-schedule

109   **$650 per pill** CTV News. (2014, May 25). Hepatitis C drugs show promise, but price is too high for most patients. www.ctvnews.ca/health/hepatitis-c-drugs-show-promise-but-price-is-too-high-for-most-patients-1.1837917

109   **$1000 per pill for a total cost of $84,000** LaMattina, J. (2014, August 8). Even at $900 (vs. $84,000 in US) Hep C cure Sovaldi's cost could be unacceptable in India. *Forbes.* http://www.forbes.com/sites/johnlamattina/2014/08/08/even-at-900-per-cure-sovaldis-cost-could-be-unacceptable-in-india/#7a804ac419a5

109   **price was set at $900** LaMattina, J. (2014, August 8). Even at $900 (vs. $84,000 in US) Hep C cure Sovaldi's cost could be unacceptable in India. *Forbes.* http://www.forbes.com/sites/johnlamattina/2014/08/08/even-at-900-per-cure-sovaldis-cost-could-be-unacceptable-in-india/#7a804ac419a5

110   **25 percent of people infected with the virus will spontaneously** Grebely, J., Raffa, J. D., Calvin, L., Krajden, M., Conway, B., & Tyndall, M. W. (2007). Factors associated with spontaneous clearance of hepatitis C virus among illicit drug users. *Canadian Journal of Gastroenterology, 21*(7), 447–451. www.ncbi.nlm.nih.gov/pmc/articles/PMC2657966

110   **In 1993, the New Zealand government introduced** Grocott, R. (2009). Applying Programme Budgeting Marginal Analysis in the health sector: 12 years of experience. *Expert Review of Pharmacoeconomics and Outcomes Research, 9*(2), 181–187. www.ncbi.nlm.nih.gov/pubmed/19402806

110   **led to savings of over $50 million** Pharmaceutical Management Agency (PHARMAC). (2016). PHARMAC tender savings top $600 million. www.pharmac.govt.nz/news/media-2015-03-17-tender-savings

112   **A recent study in Quebec found** Equale, T., Buckeridge, D. L., Winslade, N. E., Benedetti, A., Hanley, J. A., & Tamblyn, R. (2012). Drug, patient and physician characteristics associated with off-label prescribing in primary care. *Archives of Internal Medicine, 172*(10), 781–788. www.ncbi.nlm.nih.gov/pubmed/22507695

112   **Most of the solutions out there** O'Brien, M. A., Rogers, S., Jamtvedt, G., Oxman, A. D., Odgaard-Jensen, J., Kristoffersen, D. T., Forsetlund, L., Bainbridge, D., Freemantle, N., Davis, D., Haynes, R. B., & Harvey, E. (2007). Educational outreach visits: Effects on professional practice and health care outcomes. *Cochrane Database of Systematic Reviews, 4,* CD000409. www.cochrane.org/CD000409/EPOC_educational-outreach-visits-to-change-health-care-professional-care-for-patients

113   **the National Health Service maintains a "blacklist"** Mossialos, E., & Oliver, A. (2005). An overview of pharmaceutical policy in four countries: France, Germany, the Netherlands and the United Kingdom. *International Journal of*

Health Planning & Management, 20(4), 291–306. www.ncbi.nlm.nih.gov/pubmed/
16335079

113   **NHS makes these decisions according to evidence-based recommendations**
Gagnon, M-A., & Hébert, G. (2010, September 13). *The Economic Case for Universal
Pharmacare: Costs and Benefits of Publicly Funded Drug Coverage for all Canadians.*
Ottawa: Canadian Centre for Policy Alternatives. https://s3.amazonaws.com/
policyalternatives.ca/sites/default/files/uploads/publications/National%20Office/
2010/09/Universal_Pharmacare.pdf & Mossialos, E., & Oliver, A. (2005). An overview of pharmaceutical policy in four countries: France, Germany, the Netherlands
and the United Kingdom. *International Journal of Health Planning & Management,*
20(4), 291–306. www.ncbi.nlm.nih.gov/pubmed/16335079

114   **The process of academic detailing** Kondro, W. (2007). Academic drug detailing:
an evidence-based alternative. *Canadian Medical Association Journal, 176*(4), 429–431.
http://doi.org/10.1503/cmaj.070072

114   **Wise Use of Antibiotics** Pharmaceutical Management Agency. (2012). Annual
review 2012. www.pharmac.health.nz/ckeditor_assets/attachments/115/annual_
review_2012.pdf

115   **E-prescribing can also decrease prescription errors** Durieux, P., Trinquart,
L., Colombet, I., Niès, J., Walton, R., Rajeswaran, A., Rége, M. W., Harvey, E., &
Burnand, B. (2008). Computerized advice on drug dosage to improve prescribing
practice. *Cochrane Database of Systematic Reviews, 3,* CD002894. www.ncbi.nlm.
nih.gov/pubmed/18646085#

115   **effective way to improve the appropriateness of prescribing** Ivers, N.,
Jamtvedt, G., Flottorp, S., Young, J. M., Odgaard-Jensen, J., Frech, S. D., O'Brien,
M. A., Johansen, M., Grimshaw, J., & Oxman, A. D. (2012). Audit and feedback:
Effects on professional practice and healthcare outcomes. *The Cochrane Collaboration.*
http://onlinelibrary.wiley.com/doi/10.1002/14651858.CD000259.pub3/abstract

115   **despite decades of recommendations by Royal Commissions** Council of the
Federation. (2006, July 28). Council of the Federation communique. www.releases.
gov.nl.ca/releases/2006/exec/0728n05.htm

116   **A research study I was involved in** Morgan, S. G., Law, M., Daw, J. R.,
Abraham, L., & Martin, D. (2015, March 16). Estimated cost of universal public coverage of prescription drugs in Canada. *Canadian Medical Association Journal, 187*(7).
www.cmaj.ca/content/early/2015/03/16/cmaj.141564

116   **social objective of equitable access** Walkom, T. (2015). Why Canadian governments resist sensible pharmacare. *Toronto Star.* www.thestar.com/news/canada/2015/
03/17/why-canadian-governments-resist-sensible-pharmacare-walkom.html

116   **Public support for national pharmacare is high** EKOS. (2013, May 22).
Canadian views on prescription drug coverage. Press Release. www.ekospolitics.
com/wp-content/uploads/press_release_may_22_2013.pdf

116 **These economic powerhouses exert** Evans, R. (2013). Concluding Remarks. Presentation at the seminar Rethinking Drug Coverage held in Ottawa, May 25, 2013.

117 **Major change in Canadian health care is rare, but it isn't impossible** Boothe, K. (2015). *Ideas and the pace of change: National pharmaceutical insurance in Canada, Australia, and the United Kingdom.* Toronto, ON: University of Toronto Press. www.utppublishing.com/Ideas-and-the-Pace-of-Change-National-Pharmaceutical-Insurance-in-Canada-Australia-and-the-United-Kingdom.html

121 **known complication of the procedure** Werner, N., Zahn, R., & Zeymer, U. (2012, October). Stroke in patients undergoing coronary angiography and percutaneous coronary intervention: incidence, predictors, outcome and therapeutic options. *Expert Review of Cardiovascular Therapy, 10*(10), 1297–1305.

BIG IDEA 3

124 **likelihood of ending up with a Caesarean section** Alfirevic, Z., Devane, D., & Gyte, G. M. (2006). Continuous cardiotocography (CTG) as a form of electronic fetal monitoring (EFM) for fetal assessment during labour. *Cochrane Database of Systematic Reviews, 3*, CD006066. www.ncbi.nlm.nih.gov/pubmed/16856111

125 **the explosive finding in a 2015 study** Jena, A. B., Prasad, V., Godlman, D. P., & Romley, J. (2015). Mortality and treatment patterns among patients hospitalized with acute cardiovascular conditions during dates of national cardiology meetings. *Journal of the American Medical Association (JAMA) Internal Medicine, 175*(2), 237–244. http://archinte.jamanetwork.com/article.aspx?articleid=2038979

125 **In the early 2000s, a new disease known as "pre-diabetes"** Goldenberg, R., & Punthakee, Z. (2013). Definition, classification and diagnosis of diabetes, pre-diabetes and metabolic syndrome. *Canadian Journal of Diabetes, 37*, S3. www.canadianjournalofdiabetes.com/article/S1499-2671(13)00052-X/fulltext & Welch, H. G., Schwartz, L. M., & Woloshin, S. (2012). *Overdiagnosed: Making People Sick in the Pursuit of Health.* Boston: Beacon Press. www.beacon.org/Overdiagnosed-P925.aspx

126 **people with sugars below 6.0 are at increased risk** Welch, H. G., Schwartz, L. M., & Woloshin, S. (2012). *Overdiagnosed: Making People Sick in the Pursuit of Health.* Boston: Beacon Press. www.beacon.org/Overdiagnosed-P925.aspx

126 **diseases like diabetes and high blood pressure** Welch, H. G., Schwartz, L. M., & Woloshin, S. (2012). *Overdiagnosed: Making People Sick in the Pursuit of Health.* Boston: Beacon Press. www.beacon.org/Overdiagnosed-P925.aspx

126 **From a population perspective, small changes to testing thresholds** Welch, H. G., Schwartz, L. M., & Woloshin, S. (2012). *Overdiagnosed: Making People Sick in the Pursuit of Health.* Boston: Beacon Press. www.beacon.org/Overdiagnosed-P925.aspx

126   **the definition of what constitutes "abnormal" cholesterol levels** Welch, H. G., Schwartz, L. M., & Woloshin, S. (2012). *Overdiagnosed: Making People Sick in the Pursuit of Health.* Boston: Beacon Press. www.beacon.org/Overdiagnosed-P925.aspx

126   **pre-dementia, pre-diabetes, or pre-hypertension** Le Couteur, D. G., Doust, J., Creasey, H., & Brayne, C. (2013). Political drive to screen for pre-dementia: Not evidence based and ignores the harms of diagnosis. *British Medical Journal Online, 347.* www.bmj.com/content/347/bmj.f5125 & Yudkin, J. S. (2014). The epidemic of pre-diabetes: The medicine and the politics. *British Medical Journal Online, 349.* www.bmj.com/content/349/bmj.g4485

127   **A recent study looked at expert panels** Moynihan, R. N., Cooke, G. P. E., Doust, J. A., Bero, L., Hill, S., & Glasziou, P. P. (2013). Expanding disease definitions in guidelines and expert panel ties to industry: A cross-sectional study of commons conditions in the United States. *PLOS Medicine, 10*(8). http://journals.plos.org/plosmedicine/article?id=10.1371/journal.pmed.1001500.

127   **an American campaign for migraine medicine** Mintzes, B. (2006). What are the Public Health Implications? Direct-to-Consumer Advertising of Prescription Drugs in Canada. *Health Council of Canada.* www.healthcouncilcanada.ca/tree/2.38-hcc_dtc-advertising_200601_e_v6.pdf

128   **We even have a set of "ankle rules"** Stiell, I. G., Greenberg, G. H., McKnight, R. D., Nair, R. C., McDowell, I., & Worthington, J. R. (1992). A study to develop clinical decision rules for the use of radiography in acute ankle injuries. *Annals of Emergency Medicine, 21*(4), 384–390. www.ncbi.nlm.nih.gov/pubmed/1554175

128   **Our approaches to training physicians can reinforce** Weinberger, S. E. (2011). Providing high-value, cost-conscious care: A critical seventh general competency for physicians. *Annals of Internal Medicine, 155*(6), 386–388. http://annals.org/article.aspx?articleid=747128

128   **when physicians are paid for performing** Shah, B. R., Cowper, P. A., O'Brien, S. M., Jensen, N., Patel, M. R., Douglas, P. S., & Peterson, E. D. (2011). Association between physician billing and cardiac stress testing patterns following coronary revascularization. *Journal of the American Medical Association, 306*(18), 1993–2000. http://jama.jamanetwork.com/article.aspx?articleid=1104608

129   **Among the "Laws" passed down** Shem, S. (1978). *The House of God.* New York: Putnam Publishing Group, p. 361.

130   **overtesting and overtreatment are significant problems** Hicks, L. K. (2015, March 24). Reframing overuse in health care: Time to focus on the harms. *American Society of Clinical Oncology.* www.ncbi.nlm.nih.gov/pubmed/25804988

130   **The Canadian Association of Radiologists has estimated** Health Council of Canada. (2010). Decisions, decisions: Family doctors as gatekeepers to prescription drugs and diagnostic imaging in Canada. www.healthcouncilcanada.ca/tree/2.33-DecisionsHSU_Sept2010.pdf

130   **It's hard to know if this estimate is accurate** Fraser, J. (2013) Appropriateness
      of Imaging in Canada. *Canadian Association of Radiologists Journal 64*, 82–84

130   **While radiation exposure . . . is small** Peck, D. J. & Samei, E. (2010). How to
      Understand and Communicate Radiation Risk. Image Wisely. www.imagewisely.
      org/imaging-modalities/computed-tomography/medical-physicists/articles/how-to-
      understand-and-communicate-radiation-risk

131   **eliminating inappropriate CT and MRI scans** You, J. J., Levinson, W., &
      Laupacis, A. (2009). Attitudes of family physicians, specialists and radiologists
      about the use of computed tomography and magnetic resonance imaging in
      Ontario. *Health Policy, 5*(1), 54–65. www.ncbi.nlm.nih.gov/pmc/articles/
      PMC2732655/

132   **If she has a Pap smear every year** DeMay, R. M. (2000). Should we abandon
      Pap smear testing? *American Journal of Clinical Pathology, 114*(S), 48–51. www.ncbi.
      nlm.nih.gov/pubmed/11996169

132   **thousands of people are having such unnecessary screening** Kirkham, K. R.,
      Wijeysundera, D. N., Pendrith, C., Ng, R., Tu, J. V., Laupacis, A., Schull, M. J.,
      Levinson, W., & Bhatia, R. S. (2015). Preoperative testing before low-risk surgical
      procedures. *Canadian Medical Association Journal, 187*(11), E349–358. www.cmaj.
      ca/content/187/11/E349.full

133   **This unanimous recommendation is based on the fact** Simos, D., Catley, C.,
      van Walraven, C., Arnaout, A., Booth, C. M., McInnes, M., Fergusson, D., Dent, S.,
      & Clemons, M. (2015). Imaging for distant metastases in women with early-stage
      breast cancer: A population-based cohort study. *Canadian Medical Association
      Journal, 187*(12), E387–E397. www.cmaj.ca/content/early/2015/06/22/cmaj.150003

133   **a recent Ontario study** Simos, D., Catley, C., van Walraven, C., Arnaout, A.,
      Booth, C. M., McInnes, M., Fergusson, D., Dent, S., & Clemons, M. (2015). Imaging
      for distant metastases in women with early-stage breast cancer: A population-based
      cohort study. *Canadian Medical Association Journal, 187*(12), E387–E397. www.cmaj.
      ca/content/early/2015/06/22/cmaj.150003

133   **According to a newspaper article about the study** CBC News. (2015, June 22).
      Needless breast cancer imaging common in Ontario, study finds. www.cbc.ca/m/
      touch/health/story/1.3122554

134   **even three years after a false positive mammogram** Brodersen, J., & Siersma,
      V. D. (2013). Long-term psychosocial consequences of false-positive screening
      mammography. *The Annals of Family Medicine, 11*(2), 106–115. www.annfammed.org/
      content/11/2/106.full

134   **One review of all the studies on screening mammograms** Gøtzsche, P. C., &
      Jørgensen, K. (2013). Screening for breast cancer with mammography. *The Cochrane
      Library 2013*, 6. http://onlinelibrary.wiley.com/doi/10.1002/14651858.CD001877.pub5/
      abstract

135   **Dr. H. Gilbert Welch explains the problem of cancer overdiagnosis**
Welch, H. G. (2015). *Less Medicine, More Health: 7 Assumptions That Drive Too
Much Medical Care.* Boston: Beacon Press Books. www.beacon.org/Less-Medicine-
More-Health-P1095.aspx

135   **nearly 60 percent of men over the age of seventy-nine** Bell, K. J., Del Mar, C.,
Wright, G., Dickinson, J., & Glasziou, P. (2015). Prevalence of incidental prostate
cancer: A systematic review of autopsy studies. International Journal of Cancer,
137(7), 1749–1757. & Zlotta, A. R., Egawa, S., Pushkar, D., Govorov, A., Kimura, T.,
Kido, M., . . . & Fleshner, N. (2013). Prevalence of prostate cancer on autopsy: cross-
sectional study on unscreened Caucasian and Asian men. *Journal of the National
Cancer Institute, 105,* 1050–1058.

135   **likelihood that testing will turn up a "problem"** Draisma, G., Boer, R., Otto,
S. J., van der Cruijsen, I. W., Damhuis, R. A., Schröder, F. H., & de Koning, H. J.
(2003). Lead times and overdetection due to prostate-specific antigen screening:
estimates from the European Randomized Study of Screening for Prostate Cancer.
Journal of the National Cancer Institute, 95(12), 868–878.

135   **And for men who go on to have treatment for low-grade prostate cancer**
Heijnsdijk, E. A., Wever, E. M., Auvinen, A., Hugosson, J., Ciatto, S., Nelen, V., . . .
& Zappa, M. (2012). Quality-of-life effects of prostate-specific antigen screening.
New England Journal of Medicine, 367(7), 595-605.

135   **Hearing the word "cancer" understandably evokes anxiety** Welch, H. G.
(2001). Informed choice in cancer screening. *Journal of the American Medical
Association,* 285(21), 2776–2778. http://jama.jamanetwork.com/article.
aspx?articleid=193878

136   **One in four Canadians report** Ipsos R. (2015, April). Public awareness and atti-
tudes towards the Choosing Wisely campaign. Commissioned by the Canadian
Medical Association. www.choosingwiselycanada.org/news/2015/06/11/choosing-
wisely-canadas-first-birthday/

138   **Increased use of prescription medication** Canadian Institute for Health
Information. (2015). National health expenditure trends, 1975 to 2015. Data Tables,
Series G—Expenditure on drugs by type, by source of finance, by province/territory
and Canada. www.cihi.ca/en/spending-and-health-workforce/spending/national-
health-expenditure-trends

138   **In 2009 Canadian physicians wrote 80 percent more prescriptions** Health
Council of Canada. (2010). Decisions, decisions: Family doctors as gatekeepers to
prescription drugs and diagnostic imaging in Canada. www.healthcouncilcanada.ca/
tree/2.33-DecisionsHSU_Sept2010.pdf

138–   **They can be effective treatments for temporary sleep problems** Buysse, D. J.
139   (2013). Insomnia. *The Journal of the American Medical Association,* 309(7), 706–716.

139   **not supposed to be prescribed for daily use** O'Brien, Charles P. "Benzodiazepine

use, abuse, and dependence." *Journal of Clinical Psychiatry, 66*, 28–33. & Holbrook, A. M., Crowther, R., Lotter, A., Cheng, C., & King, D. (2000). Meta-analysis of benzodiazepine use in the treatment of insomnia. *Canadian Medical Association Journal, 162*(2), 225–233.

139   **should almost never be prescribed to seniors** Campanelli, C. M. (2012). American Geriatrics Society Updated Beers Criteria for Potentially Inappropriate Medication Use in Older Adults: The American Geriatrics Society 2012 Beers Criteria Update Expert Panel. *Journal of the American Geriatrics Society, 60*(4), 616–631.

139   **they're frequently prescribed these medications to help them sleep** Bell, C. M., Fischer, H. D., Gill, S. S., Zagorski, B., Sykora, K., Wodchis, W. P., . . . & Rochon, P. A. (2007). Initiation of benzodiazepines in the elderly after hospitalization. *Journal of General Internal Medicine, 22*(7), 1024–1029.

139   **Many of these people then continue being prescribed** Kermode-Scott, B. (2007). Benzodiazepine prescribing to elderly people after hospital discharge can lead to chronic use. *BMJ: British Medical Journal, 335*(7611), 119. & O'Brien, Charles P. "Benzodiazepine use, abuse, and dependence." *Journal of Clinical Psychiatry, 66*, 28–33.

139   **Sleeping pills also increase the risk of** Campanelli, C. M. (2012). American Geriatrics Society Updated Beers Criteria for Potentially Inappropriate Medication Use in Older Adults: The American Geriatrics Society 2012 Beers Criteria Update Expert Panel. *Journal of the American Geriatrics Society, 60*(4), 616–631.

139   **a group of patients receiving cataract surgery in British Columbia** Davis, J. C., McNeill, H., Wasdell, M., Chunick, S., & Bryan, S. (2012). Focussing both eyes on health outcomes: Revisiting cataract surgery. *BioMed Central Geriatrics, 12*(50). http://bmcgeriatr.biomedcentral.com/articles/10.1186/1471-2318-12-50

139   **in orthopaedic surgery, despite clear evidence** Kirkley, A., Birmingham, T. B., Litchfield, R. B., Giffin, R. J., Willits, K. R., Wong, C. J., Feagan, B. G., Donner, A., Griffin, S. H., D'Ascanio, L. M., Pope, J. E., & Fowler, P. J. (2008, September 11). A randomized trial of arthroscopic surgery for osteoarthritis of the knee. *New England Journal of Medicine, 359*, 1097–1107. www.nejm.org/doi/full/10.1056/NEJMoa0708333#t=article

140   **In the United States, it's estimated that 30 percent of all medical spending is unnecessary** Lallemand, N. C. (2012). Reducing Waste in Health Care. Health Affairs: Health Policy Brief. http://healthaffairs.org/healthpolicybriefs/brief_pdfs/healthpolicybrief_82.pdf

140   **In a 2014 survey of American physicians** Perry Undem Research/Communication. (2014). Unnecessary tests and procedures in the health care system: What physicians say about the problem, the causes, and the solutions. Results from a national survey of physicians. www.choosingwisely.org/wp-content/uploads/2014/04/042814_Final-Choosing-Wisely-Survey-Report.pdf

140   **Dr. Alberto Dolara published a call for "Slow Medicine"** Dolara, A. (2002). Invitation to "slow medicine." *Italian Heart Journal Supplement,* 3(1), 100–101. www.ncbi.nlm.nih.gov/pubmed/11899567

140   **"Slow Medicine is to health care what Slow Food is to fast food"** Slow Medicine. (2015). Slow Medicine History. www.slowmedicine.info/

140   **Economic interests, as well as cultural and social pressures** Houston, M. (2013). Welcome to Slow Medicine: Dr. Muiris Houston looks at a new concept for Irish medicine. *Medical Protection.* www.medicalprotection.org/ireland/casebook/casebook-may-2013/welcome-to-slow-medicine

141   **To achieve that culture change** American Board of Internal Medicine Foundation. (2016). Choosing Wisely: An initiative of the ABIM Foundation. www.choosingwisely.org

141   **medical groups have created** American Board of Internal Medicine Foundation. (2016). Choosing Wisely: An initiative of the ABIM Foundation. www.choosingwisely.org/clinician-lists

141   **the campaign launched in April 2014** Glauser, W. (2014). Choosing Wisely campaign well received. *Canadian Medical Association Journal, 186*(8), E239–240. www.cmaj.ca/content/186/8/E239.full

141   **at the time of writing, fifteen other countries** Choosing Wisely Canada. (2016). What is CWC? www.choosingwiselycanada.org/about/what-is-cwc/

141   **As each country develops and tests its own version** Bhatia, R. S., Levinson, W., Shortt, S., Pendrith, C., Fric-Shamji, E., Kallewaard, M., Peul, W., Veillard, J., Elshaug, A., Forde, I., & Kerr, E. A. (2015). Measuring the effect of Choosing Wisely: An integrated framework to assess campaign impact on low-value care. *British Medical Journal Quality and Safety,* 24(8). http://qualitysafety.bmj.com/content/early/2015/06/19/bmjqs-2015-004070

142   **Many others are using their information technology systems** Howell, L. P., MacDonald, S., Jones, J., Tancredi, D. J., & Melnikow, J. (2014). Can automated alerts within computerized physician order entry improve compliance with laboratory practice guidelines for ordering Pap tests? *Journal of Pathology Informatics,* 5(1), 37. www.ncbi.nlm.nih.gov/pubmed/25337434

142   **in Alberta, physicians and universities** Hnydyk, W., Cooke, L., Lang, E., & Patterson, E. (2015). Choosing Wisely Alberta & Partnerships for Implementation. www.choosingwiselycanada.org/wp-content/uploads/2015/06/Spring-Newsletter-Final.pdf

142   **At North York General Hospital in Toronto** Choosing Wisely Canada. (2015). Implementation Initiatives: North York General Hospital, Ontario, January 2015. www.choosingwiselycanada.org/resources/implementation-initiatives/2014/11/20/north-york-general-hospital-ontario-oct-2014

143   **36 percent of American physicians** Wolfson, D., Santa, J., & Slass, L. (2014).

Engaging Physicians and Consumers in Conversations About Treatment Overuse
and Waste: A Short History of the Choosing Wisely Campaign. *Academic Medicine*,
89(7), 990–995. http://journals.lww.com/academicmedicine/Fulltext/2014/07000/
Engaging_Physicians_and_Consumers_in_Conversations.17.aspx

143 **four questions that can help initiate conversations about unnecessary
care** Choosing Wisely Canada. (2015). Four Questions To Ask Your Doctor. www.
choosingwiselycanada.org/wp-content/uploads/2015/11/Four-questions-poster.pdf

144 **a decision aid can really improve** Stacey, D., Légaré, F., Col, N. F., Bennett, C. L.,
Barry, M. J., Eden, K. B., Holmes-Rovner, M., Llewellyn-Thomas, H., Lyddiatt, A.,
Thomson, R., Trevena, L., & Wu, J. H. C. (2014). Decision aids for people facing
health treatment or screening decisions. *Cochrane Database of Systematic Reviews, 1.*
https://decisionaid.ohri.ca/docs/develop/Cochrane_Review.pdf

144 **The Ottawa Hospital Research Institute** The Ottawa Hospital Research
Institute. (2015). Alphabetical list of decision aids by health topic. https://decisionaid.
ohri.ca/AZlist.html

144 **the use of decision aids has been shown** Stacey, D., Légaré, F., Col, N. F.,
Bennett, C. L., Barry, M. J., Eden, K. B., Holmes-Rovner, M., Llewellyn-Thomas, H.,
Lyddiatt, A., Thomson, R., Trevena, L., & Wu, J. H. C. (2014). Decision aids for people
facing health treatment or screening decisions. *Cochrane Database of Systematic
Reviews, Issue 1.* https://decisionaid.ohri.ca/docs/develop/Cochrane_Review.pdf

144 **the recent EMPOWER study** Tannenbaum, C., Martin, P., Tamblyn, R., Benedetti,
A., & Ahmed, S. (2014). Reduction of inappropriate benzodiazepine prescriptions
among older adults through direct patient education: The EMPOWER cluster randomized trial. *Journal of the American Medical Association (JAMA) Internal Medicine,*
174(6), 890–898. http://archinte.jamanetwork.com/article.aspx?articleid=1860498

145 **Compare this to a 5 percent success in stopping sleeping pills with our
usual approaches** Tannenbaum, C., Martin, P., Tamblyn, R., Benedetti, A., &
Ahmed, S. (2014). Reduction of inappropriate benzodiazepine prescriptions among
older adults through direct patient education: The EMPOWER cluster randomized
trial. *Journal of the American Medical Association (JAMA) Internal Medicine,* 174(6),
890–898. http://archinte.jamanetwork.com/article.aspx?articleid=1860498

BIG IDEA 4

151 **"either more of the same or actually the same with higher pay attached"**
Decter, M. (2012). Does money buy change? National Speakers Bureau, July 4, 2012.
http://nsb.com/speakers/michael-decter

152 **Improvements for dollars invested are rapid until about US$2000 in spend-
ing per capita** Organisation for Economic Co-operation and Development. (2013).
Health at a Glance 2013. www.oecd.org/els/health-systems/Health-at-a-Glance-2013.pdf

152   **we see countries like Canada spending just over CAD$6000 per capita every**
       year on health care Canadian Institute for Health Information. (2015). National
       Health Expenditure Trends, 1975 to 2015. https://secure.cihi.ca/free_products/nhex_
       trends_narrative_report_2015_en.pdf

152   **the U.S. spends almost twice as much by comparison** Organisation for
       Economic Co-operation and Development. (2015). OECD Health at a Glance 2015.
       www.keepeek.com/Digital-Asset-Management/oecd/social-issues-migration-health/
       health-at-a-glance-2015_health_glance-2015-en#page167

152   **"fix medicare for a generation"** St. Hilaire, F., & Lazar, H. (2004). A fix for a
       generation? *Policy Options.* http://policyoptions.irpp.org/issues/the-2004-federal-
       election/a-fix-for-a-generation

152   **five priority areas** Government of Canada. (2004). First minister's meeting on the
       future of health care 2004. http://healthycanadians.gc.ca/health-system-systeme-sante/
       cards-cartes/collaboration/2004-meeting-racontre-eng.php

152   **Surgical-care wait times for many procedures improved** Wait Time Alliance.
       (2015). Eliminating code gridlock in Canada's health care system: 2015 Wait Time
       Alliance report card. www.waittimealliance.ca/wp-content/uploads/2015/12/
       EN-FINAL-2015-WTA-Report-Card_REV.pdf

153   **Canadians received over four million CT scans** Health Council of Canada.
       (2010). Decisions, decisions: Family doctors as gatekeepers to prescription drugs and
       diagnostic imaging in Canada. www.healthcouncilcanada.ca/tree/2.33-DecisionsHSU_
       Sept2010.pdf

153   **less than half of the populations of P.E.I. and Alberta** Wait Time Alliance.
       (2015). Eliminating code gridlock in Canada's health care system: 2015 Wait Time
       Alliance report card. www.waittimealliance.ca/wp-content/uploads/2015/12/
       EN-FINAL-2015-WTA-Report-Card_REV.pdf

153   **at least 30 percent and up to 50 percent of imaging exams** Health Council of
       Canada. (2010). Decisions, Decisions. www.healthcouncilcanada.ca/tree/2.33-
       DecisionsHSU_Sept2010.pdf

154   **side effects including sleepiness** de Jong, M. R., Van der Elst, M., & Hartholt,
       K. A. (2013). Drug-related falls in older patients: Implicated drugs, consequences,
       and possible prevention strategies. *Therapeutic Advances in Drug Safety, 4*(4), 147–
       154. www.ncbi.nlm.nih.gov/pmc/articles/PMC4125318 & Miller, D. D. (2004).
       Atypical antipsychotics: Sleep, sedation and efficacy. *Primary Care Companion,*
       Journal of Clinical Psychiatry, 6(52), 3–7. www.ncbi.nlm.nih.gov/pmc/articles/
       PMC487011 & Schneider, L. S., Dagerman, K. S., & Insel, P. (2005). Risk of death
       with atypical antipsychotic treatment for dementia: Meta-analysis of randomized
       placebo-controlled trials. *Journal of the American Medical Association, 294*(15),
       1934–1943. http://jama.jamanetwork.com/article.aspx?articleid=201714

154   **There are other ways to control aggressive behaviour** Livingston, G., Kelly, L.,

Lewis-Holmes, E., Baio, G., Morris, S., Patel, N., Omar, R. Z., Katona, C., & Cooper, C. (2014). Non-pharmacological interventions for agitation in dementia: Systematic review of randomised controlled trials. *The British Journal of Psychiatry, 205,* 436–442. http://bjp.rcpsych.org/content/bjprcpsych/205/6/436.full.pdf

155   **it's more than two-thirds** Health Quality Ontario. (2015). Looking for balance: Antipsychotic medication use in Ontario long-term care homes. www.hqontario.ca/portals/0/Documents/pr/looking-for-balance-en.pdf

155   **survival after stroke varies substantially from province to province** Ganesh, A., Lindsay, P., Fang, J., Kapral, M. K., Côté, R., Joiner, I., Hakim, A. M., & Hill, M. D. (2016). Integrated systems of stroke care and reduction in 30-day mortality: A retrospective analysis. *Neurology, 86*(10), 898–904. www.neurology.org/content/86/10/898.short

155   **We also know that people with diabetes who live in northern or rural areas** ICES. (2012). Regional Measures of Diabetes Burden in Ontario Key Findings. www.ices.on.ca/publications/atlases-and-reports/2012/regional-measures-of-diabetes-burden-in-ontario & World Diabetes Foundation. (2014). Prevention of Blindness WDF07-275. http://www.worlddiabetesfoundation.org/projects/india-wdf07-275

155   **Women with invasive breast cancer in Newfoundland** Canadian Institute for Health Information. (2012). Breast Cancer Surgery in Canada, 2007–2008 to 2009–2010. https://secure.cihi.ca/free_products/BreastCancer_7-8_9-10_EN.pdf

156   **nearly one-quarter of our country's population will be over sixty-five** Government of Canada. (2016). Canada's Aging Population. http://publications.gc.ca/collections/Collection/H39-608-2002E.pdf

156   **seniors represented 19 percent of the population of Nova Scotia** Statistics Canada. (2015). Chart 4: Proportion of the population aged 0 to 14 years and 65 years and older, July 1, 2015, Canada, provinces and territories. www.statcan.gc.ca/daily-quotidien/150929/cg-b004-eng.htm

156   **as people age and live longer with multiple chronic diseases** Canadian Institute for Health Information. (2011). Seniors and the health care system: What is the impact of multiple chronic conditions? https://secure.cihi.ca/free_products/air-chronic_disease_aib_en.pdf

156   **Only one in four Canadian seniors with a chronic condition** Canadian Institute for Health Information. (2011). Seniors and the health care system: What is the impact of multiple chronic conditions? https://secure.cihi.ca/free_products/air-chronic_disease_aib_en.pdf

157   **97 percent of seniors are satisfied** Public Health Agency of Canada. (2010). The Chief Public Health Officer's report on the state of public health in Canada. Table 3.2: Health of Canada's seniors. www.phac-aspc.gc.ca/cphorsphc-respcacsp/2010/fr-rc/cphorsphc-respcacsp-06-eng.php

157– *the highest numbers of new Canadians came from the Philippines, China,*
158   *and India* Immigration, Refugees, and Citizenship Canada. (2011). Facts and fig-
      ures—Immigration overview. Permanent and temporary residents. www.cic.gc.ca/
      english/resources/statistics/facts2011/permanent/10.asp

158   *heart disease, high blood pressure, and diabetes* Chiu, M., Austin, P. C.,
      Manuel, D. G., & Tu, J. V. (2010). Comparison of cardiovascular risk profiles among
      ethnic groups using population health surveys between 1996 and 2007. *Canadian
      Medical Association Journal, 182*(8), E301–310. www.cmaj.ca/content/182/8/E301.abstract

158   *first-generation immigrant adults are generally healthier* Vang, Z., Sigouin, J.,
      Flenon, A., & Gagnon, M-A. (2015). The healthy immigrant effect in Canada: A
      systematic review. *Population Change and Lifecourse Strategic Knowledge Cluster
      Discussion Paper Series, 3*(1). http://ir.lib.uwo.ca/cgi/viewcontent.cgi?article=1012
      &context=pclc

158   *"Instead of just looking up symptoms . . ."* Sifferlin, A. (2015, September 10).
      Here's what 6 doctors really think of Dr. Google. *Time.* http://time.com/4025756/
      google-health-issues-doctor

159   *Let Patients Help! is a manifesto for participatory medicine* deBronkart, Jr.,
      R. D. (2013). *Let Patients Help! A patient engagement handbook.* CreateSpace
      Independent Publishing Platform. www.epatientdave.com/let-patients-help/

159   *a generation to completely arrive at a new reality* e-Patient Dave. (2015).
      Berci's "My Health: Upgraded": A futurist vision worthy of Doc Tom. www.
      epatientdave.com/2015/09/22/bercis-my-health-upgraded-a-futurist-vision-worthy-
      of-doc-tom/#more-10646

159   *appropriate use of less expensive and more empowering self-care*
      deBronkart, D. (2013). How the e-patient community helped save my life: An essay by
      Dave deBronkart. *British Medical Journal, 346.* www.bmj.com/content/346/bmj.f1990

160   *Something as simple as a chair can make a big difference* Glouberman, S.
      (2014). Small changes with impact: The third chair in triage. https://
      healthandeverythingblog.wordpress.com/2014/09/10/minimal-interventions-a-third-
      chair-in-triage

160   *our spending is concentrated among a small group of people* Rais, S.,
      Nazerian, A., Ardal, S., Chechulin, Y., Bains, N., & Malikov, K. (2013). High-cost
      users of Ontario's healthcare services. *Healthcare Policy, 9*(1), 44–51. www.ncbi.nlm.
      nih.gov/pubmed/23968673

160   *1 percent of the province's health care users* Deber, R. B., & Lam, K. C. K.
      (2009). Handling the high spenders: Implications of the distribution of health
      expenditures for financing health care. Paper presented at the 2009 American
      Political Science Association Annual Meeting, Toronto, Canada. http://papers.ssrn.
      com/sol3/papers.cfm?abstract_id=1450788

161   *in Ontario, only 45 percent remained in that category* Wodchis, W. P.,

Austin, P. C., & Henry, D. A. (2016). A 3-year study of high-cost users of health care. *Canadian Medical Association Journal, 188*(3), 182–188. www.cmaj.ca/content/early/2016/01/11/cmaj.150064

161 **people whose high-intensity needs are chronic** Canadian Institute for Health Information. (2011). Seniors and the health care system: What is the impact of multiple chronic conditions? https://secure.cihi.ca/free_products/air-chronic_disease_aib_en.pdf

161 **others are frail, medically complex, or have a severe, relapsing condition** Vaillancourt, S., Shahin, I., Aggarwal, P., Pomedli, S., Hayden, L., Pus, L., & Bhattacharyya, O. (2014, July). Using archetypes to design services for high users of health care. *Healthcare Papers, 14*(2), 37–41. www.ncbi.nlm.nih.gov/pubmed/25880862

161 **In Canada, one in every twelve hospitalized patients** Canadian Institute for Health Information. (2012). All-cause readmission to acute care and return to the emergency department. https://secure.cihi.ca/free_products/Readmission_to_acutecare_en.pdf

161 **in the U.S., it's one in eight** Tsai, T. C., Joynt, K. E., Orav, J., Gawande, A. A., & Jha, A. K. (2013). Variation in surgical-readmission rates and quality of hospital care. *New England Journal of Medicine, 369,* 1134–1142. www.nejm.org/doi/full/10.1056/NEJMsa1303118

163 **when I refer a patient with late-stage osteoarthritis of the knee.** Sunnybrook Health Sciences Centre. (2007). New Assessment Model for Hip and Knee Replacement. http://sunnybrook.ca/uploads/MSK_AssessHKR.pdf

166 **among the lowest number of beds per capita** Organisation for Economic Co-operation and Development. (2014). Hospital beds: Density per 1,000 population. www.oecd-ilibrary.org/social-issues-migration-health/hospital-beds_20758480-table5; jsessionid=33dmec807jdht.x-oecd-live-03

167 **primary health care, home care, . . . and rehabilitation** Decter, M. (2014). Saving medicare: As costs steadily rise, we need to build a healthcare system outside hospitals. http://reviewcanada.ca/magazine/2014/09/saving-medicare

167– **They're solo practitioners, or they work in small groups of two or three**
168 **doctors** SCOPE Project. Unpublished data.

168 **project called SCOPE** University Hospital Network. (2016). About SCOPE. www.uhn.ca/healthcareprofessionals/SCOPE

168 **method known as hot-spotting** Gawande, A. (2011, January). The Hotspotters. *The New Yorker.* www.newyorker.com/magazine/2011/01/24/the-hot-spotters

171 **cheaper, simpler, or more convenient** Christensen, C. M., Bohmer, R. M. J., & Kenagy, J. (2000). Will disruptive innovations cure health care? *Harvard Business Review.* https://hbr.org/2000/09/will-disruptive-innovations-cure-health-care

171 **gaining a foothold by doing things in a way** Christensen, C. M., Raynor, M. E., & McDonald, R. (2015, December). What is disruptive innovation? *Harvard Business Review.* https://hbr.org/2015/12/what-is-disruptive-innovation

172   **during a three-year research trial** Ontario Telemedicine Network (OTN). (2013). Case study—telemedicine: A tool for the rehabilitation and socialization of stroke patients in remote communities. https://otn.ca/sites/default/files/otn-telemedicine-case-study-taylor.pdf

174   **The PATH clinic in Nova Scotia** PATH Clinic. (2013). About PATH: What is PATH? www.pathclinic.ca/getting_started

174   **most Canadians want to die either at home or in some other safe, comfortable, non-hospital setting** Canadian Institute for Health Information. (2007). Health care use at the end of life in western Canada. Ottawa: CIHI, p. 22. https://secure.cihi.ca/free_products/end_of_life_report_aug07_e.pdf

174   **more than half of all deaths occur in hospital** Statistics Canada. (2012). Table 102-0509: Deaths in hospital and elsewhere, Canada, provinces and territories. www5.statcan.gc.ca/cansim/a26?lang=eng&id=1020509

175   **from providing care "to patients"** Balik, B. (2015). To—for—with: The journey to understanding partnerships with patients. www.changefoundation.ca/library/barbara-balik-to-for-with-the-journey-to-understanding-partnerships-with-patients

176   **Consider the Northumberland Hills Hospital** Canadian Institutes of Health Research. (2013). Case 6: Shared challenge, shared solution: Northumberland Hills Hospital's collaborative budget strategy. www.cihr-irsc.gc.ca/e/47593.html & Northumberland Hills Hospital. (2010, January). Citizens' Advisory Panel on Health Service Prioritization, final report. www.nhh.ca/LinkClick.aspx?fileticket=jpyxIoXLcDQ%3D&tabid=587&language=en-US

177   **We used to say that 50 percent of startups fail** Noble, C. (2011). Why Companies Fail—and How Their Founders Can Bounce Back. *Harvard Business School Working Knowledge.* http://hbswk.hbs.edu/item/why-companies-failand-how-their-founders-can-bounce-back

177   **John Maxwell even wrote a whole book** Maxwell, J. (2000). *Failing Forward: Turning Mistakes into Stepping Stones for Success.* Nashville: Thomas Nelson, Inc. https://books.google.ca/books?id=FzCNE9j4u1MC&printsec=frontcover&source=gbs_ge_summary_r&cad=0#v=onepage&q&f=false

178   **targeted at patients who were being discharged from hospital** Singer, H. (2014, Fall). From hospital to home: Closing the cracks in care. *U of T Medicine.* Toronto: University of Toronto Faculty of Medicine. www.facmed.utoronto.ca/magazine/article/hospital-home-closing-cracks-care

178   **the results of the evaluation were disappointing** Dhalla, I. A., O'Brien, T., Morra, D., Thorpe, K. E., Wong, B. M., Mehta, R., Frost, D. W., Abrams, H., Ko, F., Van Rooyen, P., Bell, C. M., Gruneir, A., Lewis, G. H., Daub, S., Anderson, G. M., Hawker, G. A., Rochon, P. A., & Laupacis, A. (2014). Effect of a Postdischarge Virtual Ward on Readmission or Death for High-Risk Patients: A Randomized

Clinical Trial. *The Journal of the American Medical Association*, 312(13), 1305-1312. http://jama.jamanetwork.com/article.aspx?articleid=1910109

179 **According to the business literature** O'Reilly, Charles A. and Tushman, Michael L. (2004). The ambidextrous organization. *Harvard Business Review, April*: 74–83.

179 **So we're increasingly monitoring handwashing rates** Health Quality Ontario and ICES. (2012). Report on Ontario's Health System. www.hqontario.ca/portals/o/documents/pr/qmonitor-full-report-2012-en.pdf

180 **EWB publishes a Failure Report** Engineers Without Borders Canada. (2011). Failure Report. legacy.ewb.ca/en/whoweare/accountable/failure.html

182 **more support than just education** Bhattacharyya, O., Hayden, L., & Hensel, J. (2015, June 2). Health services and designing for uncertainty. *Stanford Social Innovation Review*, Health. http://ssir.org/articles/entry/health_services_and_designing_for_uncertainty

BIG IDEA 5

188 **Leslie wasn't sick with asthma. She was sick with poverty** Meili, Ryan. Personal correspondence.

189 **income is the strongest predictor of health** Canadian Medical Association. (2015). Health equity and the social determinants of health. www.cma.ca/En/Pages/health-equity.aspx

189 **Canadians are more likely to die at an earlier** The Federal, Provincial and Territorial Advisory Committee on Population Health. (1999). Towards a healthy future: A second report on the health of Canadians. Prepared for the Meeting of Ministers of Health, Charlottetown, P.E.I., September 1999. http://publications.gc.ca/collections/Collection/H39-468-1999E.pdf

189 **income affects health indirectly** Marmot, M. (2002). The influence of income on health: Views of an epidemiologist. *Health Affairs, 21*(2), 31–46. http://content.healthaffairs.org/content/21/2/31.full.pdf+html?sid=2475f44b-f40c-402c-8c27-149a5008fdfe

189 **You are standing on the edge of a river . . .** Upstream. (2013). Introduction to Upstream. Online video clip. www.thinkupstream.net/about_upstream

190 **the social determinants of health** Canadian Institute for Advanced Research, Health Canada, Population and Public Health Branch AB/NWT. (2002). Estimated impact of determinants on health status of the population. www.thinkupstream.net/anniversary_blog_charles_plante

191 **Poverty has an effect on health** Currie, J. (2008). *Healthy, Wealthy and Wise: Socioeconomic Status, Poor Health in Childhood, and Human Capital Development*. Working Paper 13987. Boston: National Bureau of Economic Research. http://web.stanford.edu/group/scspi/_media/pdf/Reference%20Media/Currie_2008_Health%20and%20Mental%20Health.pdf

191   *These differences are apparent in lower birth weights* Paul-Sen Gupta, R.,
       de Wit, M. L., & McKeown, D. (2007, October). The impact of poverty on the current
       and future health status of children. *Paediatrics and Child Health, 12*(8), 667–672.
       www.ncbi.nlm.nih.gov/pmc/articles/PMC2528796/pdf/pch12667.pdf

192   *They may move into low-cost housing* Fransoo, R., Martens, P., The Need to Know
       Team, Prior, H., Burchill, C., Koseva, I., Bailly, A., & Allegro, E. (2013, October). The
       2013 RHA Indicators Atlas. Winnipeg: Manitoba Centre for Health Policy, Department
       of Community Health Sciences, Faculty of Medicine, University of Manitoba.
       http://mchp-appserv.cpe.umanitoba.ca/reference//RHA_2013_web_version.pdf

192   *This is the part of the city* PEG. (2015). Our city: A PEG report on health equity.
       www.mypeg.ca/sites/default/files/uploads/Peg%20Health%20Equity%20Report%20
       -%20FINAL.pdf

192   *Those kinds of risk factors* Laurie, N. Drummond, D., Maxwell, J., Milway, J.
       Stabile, M., Stapleton, J., Spence, A., Park, S., Bednar, V., Murphy, J., Suave, R.,
       Barata, P., & Murphy, C. (2008, November). The cost of poverty: An analysis of the
       economic cost of poverty in Ontario. https://ccednet-rcdec.ca/sites/ccednet-rcdec.ca/
       files/ccednet/pdfs/2008-OAFB-Cost_of_Poverty_in_Ontario.pdf

192   *If you live in Ontario, poverty costs your household* Laurie, N. Drummond,
       D., Maxwell, J., Milway, J., Stabile, M., Stapleton, J., Spence, A., Park, S., Bednar,
       V., Murphy, J., Suave, R., Barata, P., & Murphy, C. (2008, November). The cost of
       poverty: An analysis of the economic cost of poverty in Ontario. https://ccednet-
       rcdec.ca/sites/ccednet-rcdec.ca/files/ccednet/pdfs/2008-OAFB-Cost_of_Poverty_
       in_Ontario.pdf

192   *estimated cost of poverty in Saskatchewan* Plante, C., & Sharp, K. (2014,
       October). Poverty costs Saskatchewan: A new approach to prosperity for all.
       Saskatoon: Poverty Costs. https://d3n8a8pro7vhmx.cloudfront.net/upstream/pages/241/
       attachments/original/1416962412/poverty-costs-sk-summary-2014.pdf?1416962412

193   *In their book* The Spirit Level: Why Greater Equality Makes Societies
       Stronger Wilkinson, R. G., & Pickett, K. (2009). *The Spirit Level: Why Greater
       Equality Makes Societies Stronger.* Bloomsbury Press.

193   *the current rate in Newfoundland for a couple* Government of Newfoundland
       and Labrador. (2015). Department of Advanced Education and Skills. Program
       Overview. www.aes.gov.nl.ca/income-support/overview.html

193   *the average monthly rent for a two-bedroom apartment* Canada Mortgage
       and Housing Corporation. (2015, Spring). Rental market report: Newfoundland and
       Labrador highlights. www.cmhc-schl.gc.ca/odpub/esub/64499/64499_2015_B01.pdf

194   *"deeply inefficient, fraught with bureaucratic excess . . ."* Segal, H. (2013,
       June 8). Why guaranteeing the poor an income will save us all in the end. *The
       Huffington Post.* www.huffingtonpost.ca/hugh-segal/guaranteed-annual-
       income_b_3037347.html

Citations 285

194   **People on social assistance** Torjman, S., & Battle, K. (1993, July). Breaking down the welfare wall. *The Caledon Institute of Social Policy.* www.caledoninst.org/Publications/PDF/488ENG.pdf

194   **Moreover, if a mother finds a job for minimum wage** Segal, H. (2012, December). Scrapping Welfare: The case for guaranteeing all Canadians an income above the poverty line. *Literary Review of Canada.* http://reviewcanada.ca/magazine/2012/12/scrapping-welfare/

194   **"Our present system . . ."** Segal, Hugh. (2012). Scrapping Welfare. The case for guaranteeing all Canadians an income above the poverty line. *Literary Review Canada.* reviewcanada.ca/magazine/2012/12/scrapping-welfare

196   **Basic Income Guarantee can't and mustn't replace all social programs** Advisory Group on Poverty Reduction. (2015). Recommendations for a provincial poverty reduction strategy. www.saskatchewan.ca/~/media/news%20release%20backgrounders/2015/aug/advisory%20group%20on%20poverty%20reduction%20report.pdf

197   **"would not be treated as dim creatures . . ."** Segal, H. (2012, December). Scrapping welfare: The case for guaranteeing all Canadians an income above the poverty line. *Literary Review of Canada.* http://reviewcanada.ca/magazine/2012/12/scrapping-welfare

199   **The guaranteed annual income works** Simpson, W. (2012). Guaranteed Annual Income (GAI), Basic Income (BI) and the Manitoba Basic Annual Income Experiment (Mincome). http://winnipegharvest.org/wp-content/uploads/2012/08/Presentation-by-Wayne-Simpson-on-Guaranteed-Annual-Income.pptx

200   **Most versions that currently exist** Hellmann, A. G. (2015, September). How does Bolsa Familia work? Best practices in the implementation of conditional cash transfer programs in Latin America and the Caribbean. *Inter-American Development Bank.* https://publications.iadb.org/bitstream/handle/11319/7210/How_does_Bolsa_Familia_Work.pdf?sequence=5

200   **we may see a universal cash transfer** Kansaneläkelaitos: The Social Insurance Institution of Finland (Kela). (2015). Contrary to reports, basic income study still at preliminary stage. www.kela.fi/web/en/press-releases/-/asset_publisher/LgL2IQBbkg98/content/contrary-to-reports-basic-income-study-still-at-preliminary-stage

201   **The Dutch city of Utrecht** Boffey, D. (2015). Dutch city plans to pay citizens a 'basic income', and Greens say it could work in the UK. *The Guardian.* www.theguardian.com/world/2015/dec/26/dutch-city-utrecht-basic-income-uk-greens

201   **In the 1960s and 1970s** Forget, E. (2015, October). Reconsidering a Guaranteed Annual Income: Lessons from MINCOME. *Public Sector Digest, Economics and Finance.* www.publicsectordigest.com/articles/view/1506

201   **South of our border, building on the momentum** Hyndman, B., & Simon, L. (2015, October). Basic Income Guarantee: Backgrounder. www.opha.on.ca/getmedia/

bf22640d-120c-46db-ac69-315fb9aa3c7c/alPHa-OPHA-HEWG-Basic-Income-
Backgrounder-Final-Oct-2015.pdf.aspx?ext=.pdf

201   **They called the experiment Mincome** Forget, E. (2015, October). Reconsidering
a Guaranteed Annual Income: Lessons from MINCOME. *Public Sector Digest:
Economics and Finance.* www.publicsectordigest.com/articles/view/1506

203   **Before Mincome came along** Forget, E. (2015, October). Reconsidering a
Guaranteed Annual Income: Lessons from MINCOME. *Public Sector Digest:
Economics and Finance.* www.researchgate.net/publication/282878565_

204   **The effects extended beyond health services** Forget, E. L. (2011). The Town
With No Poverty: Using Health Administration Data to Revisit Outcomes of a
Canadian Guaranteed Annual Income Field Experiment. *University of Manitoba.*
http://nccdh.ca/images/uploads/comments/forget-cea_(2).pdf

204   **On the other side of the world** Remme, M., Vassall, A., Lutz, B., Luna, J., &
Watts, C. (2014). Financing structural interventions: Going beyond HIV-only value
for money assessments. *AIDS, 28,* 425–434. www.unicef.org/tanzania/Remme_et_al._
2014._Financingstructural_interventions_-_going_beyond_HIV-only_value_for_
moneyassessments.pdf

204   **Some received this money** Baird, S. J., Garfein, R. S., McIntosh, C. T., & Özler, B.
(2012, April). Effect of a cash transfer programme for schooling on prevalence of HIV
and herpes simplex type 2 in Malawi: A cluster randomised trial. *The Lancet,
379*(9823), 1320–1329. www.sciencedirect.com/science/article/pii/S0140673611617091

205   **As Hugh Segal tells the story** Segal, H. (2014). Senator speaks about guaranteed
annual income. Toronto: Anglican Church of Canada. www.toronto.anglican.
ca/2014/05/26/senator-speaks-about-guaranteed-annual-income-at-church

205   **Today, all Canadian seniors** Emery, J. C., Fleisch, V. C., & McIntyre, L. (2013,
December). Legislated changes to federal pension income in Canada will adversely
affect low income seniors' health. *Preventive Medicine, 57*(6), 963–966. www.ncbi.
nlm.nih.gov/pubmed/24055151

205   **Food insecurity drops from 23 percent** Emery, J. C., Fleisch, V. C., & McIntyre,
L. (2013, December). Legislated changes to federal pension income in Canada will
adversely affect low income seniors' health. *Preventive Medicine, 57*(6), 963–966.
www.ncbi.nlm.nih.gov/pubmed/24055151

205   **At the other end of the age spectrum** Simpson, W. (2015, June). Basic income,
guaranteed income and tax credits: What's the difference? *University of Calgary
School of Public Policy.* http://policyschool.ucalgary.ca/?q=content/basic-income-
guaranteed-income-and-tax-credits-what's-difference

205   **Families that receive the child benefit** Milligan, K., & Stabile, M. (2011, August).
Do child tax benefits affect the well-being of children? Evidence from Canadian
child benefit expansions. *American Economic Journal: Economic Policy, 3*(3), 175–205.
http://courses.washington.edu/pbafadv/examples/child%20benefit%20IV.pdf

205   **around one-third of the Canadian population** Broadway, Robin. Personal
       correspondence.

205–   **If one were to use the 2016 Low Income Cut-Off** Citizenship and Immigration
206   Canada. (2016). Applying for a Visitor Visa (Temporary Resident Visa—IMM 5256)
       Income Table. www.cic.gc.ca/english/information/applications/guides/
       5256ETOC.asp#incometables & Statistics Canada. (2015). Low income cut-offs.
       www.statcan.gc.ca/pub/75fooo2m/2012002/lico-sfr-eng.htm

206   **According to some estimates** Goar, C. (2015, March). National income floor for
       troubled times: Goar. *Toronto Star*. www.thestar.com/opinion/commentary/2015/
       03/08/national-income-floor-for-troubled-times-goar.html & Segal, H. (2012).
       Scrapping welfare: The case for guaranteeing all Canadians an income above the
       poverty line. *Literary Review of Canada*. http://reviewcanada.ca/magazine/2012/12/
       scrapping-welfare

206   **Other estimates have ranged from** National Council of Welfare. (2011). The
       dollars and sense of poverty. http://publications.gc.ca/collections/collection_2011/
       cnb-ncw/HS54-2-2011-eng.pdf & Roos, N., & Forget, E. (2015, August 4). The time
       for a guaranteed annual income might finally have come. *The Globe and Mail*. www.
       theglobeandmail.com/report-on-business/rob-commentary/the-time-for-a-guaranteed-
       annual-income-might-finally-have-come/article25819266/ß

206   **The relief gained by so many other spending areas** Laurie, N., Drummond,
       D., Maxwell, J., Milway, J. Stabile, M., Stapleton, J., Spence, A., Park, S., Bednar,
       V., Murphy, J., Suave, R., Barata, P., & Murphy, C. (2008, November). The cost of
       poverty: An analysis of the economic cost of poverty in Ontario. https://ccednet-
       rcdec.ca/sites/ccednet-rcdec.ca/files/ccednet/pdfs/2008-OAFB-Cost_of_Poverty_
       in_Ontario.pdf

206   **In Namibia, with a basic income, self-employment jumped 300 percent**
       Basic Income Earth Network. (2013). NewsFlash. *NewsFlash* 26 (70). & Krozer, A.
       (2010). A Regional Basic Income: Towards the Eradication of Extreme Poverty in
       Central America. *CEPAL*. repositorio.cepal.org/bitstream/11362/25938/1/lcmexl998.
       pdf & UNICEF. (2012). Transformative Transfers: Evidence from Liberia's Social
       Cash Transfer Programme. http://www.unicef.org/liberia/Transformative_Transfers_
       LiberiaCashTransferProgramme.pdf

206–   **As columnist Andrew Coyne has pointed out** Coyne, A. (2015, June 10).
207   Guarantee a minimum income, not a minimum wage. *National Post*. http://news.
       nationalpost.com/full-comment/andrew-coyne-guarantee-a-minimum-income-not-a-
       minimum-wage

207   **Yet in Brazil, families spend the money** Guanais, F. (2011). Bolsa Familia pro-
       gram, funding families for development: A case study. *NS World*. www.pgionline.com/
       wp-content/uploads/2015/08/Bolsa-Fam%C3%ADlia-Program-Funding-Families-for-
       Development.pdf

207   **In Kenya, when people living in poverty were given** Reuters. (2015, May 11).
       Cash aid feeds business surge in northeast Kenya. www.reuters.com/article/2015/05/
       11/us-kenya-aid-idUSKBN0NW0C120150511

207   **Would low-income Canadians spend a basic income on beer and popcorn**
       CBC News. (2005). Liberal apologizes for saying Harper day-care bucks may buy
       beer, popcorn. http://www.cbc.ca/news/canada/liberal-apologizes-for-saying-harper-
       day-care-bucks-may-buy-beer-popcorn-1.534811

207   **Researcher Mark Stabile at the University of Toronto and his colleagues**
       Jones, L., Milligan, K., & Stabile, M. (2015, March). How do families who receive the
       CCTB and NTB spend the money? http://martinprosperity.org/media/CCTB-and-
       NCB-Family-Spending.pdf

207   **"almost without exception, studies find . . ."** Evans, D. K., & Popova, A.
       (2014, May). Cash transfer and temptation goods: A review of global evidence. Policy
       Research Working Paper 6886. *Africa Region, Office of the Chief Economist: The
       World Bank.* www-wds.worldbank.org/external/default/WDSContentServer/IW3P/
       IB/2014/05/21/000158349_20140521143938/Rendered/PDF/WPS6886.pdf

207   **mothers in the U.S. who received a cash supplement** Hoynes, H., Miller, D., &
       David, S. (2015). Income, the earned income tax credit, and infant health. *American
       Economic Journal: Economic Policy, 7*(1), 172–211. www.nber.org/papers/w18206.pdf

208   **The Basic Income Guarantee idea is catching on** Segal, H. (2013, April 8).
       Why guaranteeing the poor an income will save us all in the end. *The Huffington
       Post.* www.huffingtonpost.ca/hugh-segal/guaranteed-annual-income_b_3037347.html

208   **Liberals, Conservatives, New Democrats, and the Greens** Blanchard, M.
       (2014). Time to move to basic income guarantee. *New Democratic Party of Prince
       Edward Island.* www.ndppei.ca/time-to-move-to-basic-income-guarantee & Green
       Party of Canada. (2015). Vision Green 2015. www.greenparty.ca/sites/default/files/
       vision_green_2015_-_updated_august_2015_-_reduced.pdf & Liberal Party of
       Canada. (2015). 97. Basic income supplement: Testing a dignified approach to
       income security for working-age Canadians. www.liberal.ca/policy-resolutions/97-
       basic-income-supplement-testing-dignified-approach-income-security-workingage-
       canadians & Liberal Party of Canada. (2015). 100. Priority resolution: Creating a
       basic annual income to be designated and implemented for a fair economy. www.
       liberal.ca/policy-resolutions/100-priority-resolution-creating-basic-annual-income-
       designed-implemented-fair-economy

208   **Mayors from all over Canada** Benns, R. (2015, November 2). All three northern
       capital city mayors say it's time to look at basic income. http://leadersandlegacies.
       com/2015/11/02/all-three-northern-capital-city-mayors-say-its-time-to-look-at-basic-
       income & Benns, R. (2015, September 28). Mayors of St. Catharines, Niagara Falls
       declare support for basic income. http://leadersandlegacies.com/2015/09/28/mayors-of-
       st-catharines-niagara-falls-declare-support-for-basic-income & King, R. L. (2015, June 5).

Alberta mayors back guaranteed minimum income. *Toronto Star*. www.thestar.com/news/canada/2015/06/05/alberta-mayors-stick-back-guaranteed-minimum-income.html

BIG IDEA 6

211   **Every time a kidney is transplanted** The Kidney Foundation of Canada. (2012). Facing the facts. www.kidney.ca/facing-the-facts

212   **the Highly Sensitized Patient program** Canadian Blood Services. (2015, May 22). New program will improve chances of a kidney transplant for hard-to-match patients. News release. www.blood.ca/en/media/new-program-will-improve-chances-kidney-transplant-hard-match-patients

213   **Canadians who require stem-cell transplantation** Canadian Blood Services. (2015, June 25). News release. Canadian Blood Services' Cord Blood Bank is now officially launched. www.blood.ca/en/media/canadian-blood-services-cord-blood-bank-is-now-officially-launched

213   **a groundbreaking program that helps** Moorhouse, P., & Mallery, L. (2010). PATH: A new approach to end-of-life care. *The Canadian Review of Alzheimer's Disease and Other Dementias*, 4–8. www.stacommunications.com/customcomm/Back-issue_pages/AD_Review/adPDFs/2010/May2010/04.pdf

213   **reduce wait times for hip and knee replacements** Alberta's physicians and health regions, Alberta Health and Wellness, & Alberta Bone and Joint Institute. (2008). An Innovative Made-in-Alberta Model for Hip and Knee Replacements. www.albertaboneandjoint.com/wp-content/uploads/2013/12/At-A-Glance_12_Mo_Pilot_Results_March_08_Final.pdf

213   **"the single biggest problem . . ."** Lewis, S. (2007). Commentary. *Healthcare Quarterly, 10*(2), 103–104. www.longwoods.com/content/18840

214   **If you want a project to spread beyond the local** Mittman, B. (2014). Factors that influence the scale up and spread of innovations. *Agency for Healthcare Research and Quality, Health Care Innovations Exchange*. https://innovations.ahrq.gov/perspectives/factors-influence-scale-and-spread-innovations

216   **the World Health Organization's surgical safety checklist** World Health Organization. (2009). WHO guidelines for safe surgery: Safe surgery saves lives. http://apps.who.int/iris/bitstream/10665/44185/1/9789241598552_eng.pdf

216   **They confirm the patient's identity** Urbach, D. R., Govindarajan, A., Saskin, R., Wilton, A. S., & Baxter, N. N. (2014). Adoption of surgical safety checklists in Ontario, Canada: Overpromised or underdelivered? *Healthcare Quarterly, 17*(4). www.longwoods.com/content/24125

217   **the risk of that person dying decreases by roughly 50 percent** Haynes, A. B., Weiser, T. G., Berry, W. R., Lipsitz, S. R., Breizat, A. S., Dellinger, P., Herbosa, T., Joseph, S., Kibatala, P. L., Lapitan, M. C. M., Merry, A. F., Moorthy, K., Reznick, R. K.,

Taylor, B., & Gawande, A. A. (2009). A surgical safety checklist to reduce morbidity and mortality in a global population. *New England Journal of Medicine, 360*(5), 491–499. www.nejm.org/doi/full/10.1056/NEJMsa0810119

217   *Very few health care improvement projects get implemented* Naylor, David, Girard, Francine, Fraser, Neil, Jenkins, Toby, Mintz, Jack & Power, Christine. (2014). Unleashing Innovation: Excellent Healthcare for Canada. Report of the Advisory Panel on Healthcare Innovation. www.healthycanadians.gc.ca/publications/health-system-systeme-sante/report-healthcare-innovation-rapport-soins/alt/report-healthcare-innovation-rapport-soins-eng.pdf

217   *"seven spreadly sins"* Institute for Healthcare Improvement. (2015). Seven spreadly sins. Infographic. Cambridge, Massachusetts. www.ihi.org/resources/pages/tools/ihisevenspreadlysins.aspx

218   *They studied 101 hospitals* Urbach, D. R., Govindarajan, A., Saskin, R., Wilton, A. S., & Baxter, N. N. (2014). Introduction of surgical safety checklists in Ontario, Canada. *The New England Journal of Medicine, 370*(11), 1029–1038. www.nejm.org/doi/pdf/10.1056/NEJMsa1308261

218   *When a pilot project succeeds in one environment* Plsek, P. E. & Associates, Inc. (2015). Creating a culture of innovation. *Agency for Healthcare Research and Quality, Health Care Innovations Exchange.* https://innovations.ahrq.gov/article/creating-culture-innovation

220   *the time to the "third next available" appointment* Institute for Healthcare Improvement. (2015). Third next available appointment. www.ihi.org/resources/Pages/Measures/ThirdNextAvailableAppointment.aspx

220   *the team secretary starts offering you appointment times* Institute for Healthcare Improvement. (2015) Third next available appointment. www.ihi.org/resources/Pages/Measures/ThirdNextAvailableAppointment.aspx

221   *When audit and feedback inspire change* Ivers, N., Jamtvedt, G., Flottorp, S., Young, J. M., Odgaard-Jensen, J., Frech, S. D., O'Brien, M. A., Johansen, M., Grimshaw, J., & Oxman, A. D. (2012). Audit and feedback: Effects on professional practice and patient outcomes. *The Cochrane Collaboration.* http://onlinelibrary.wiley.com/doi/10.1002/14651858.CD000259.pub3/abstract;jsessionid=C89E463DA632A3B6F8B3F8E74DA14321.f02t03

221   *While those tricks don't solve everything* Kiran, T., & O'Brien, P. (2015). Challenge of same-day access in primary care. *Canadian Family Physician, 61*(5), 399–400. www.cfp.ca/content/61/5/399.full

223   *In the U.S., the Centers for Medicare* Centers for Medicare & Medicaid Services. (2016). Hospital Compare. www.medicare.gov/hospitalcompare/search.html

223   *the Canadian Institute for Health Information launched a much less detailed* Canadian Institute for Health Information. (2016). Explore Your Health System. http://yourhealthsystem.cihi.ca/hsp/indepth?lang=en

223   **websites don't always convey information that matters** Jha, A. K. (2015). Health care providers should publish physician ratings. *Harvard Business Review: Assessing Performance.* https://hbr.org/2015/10/health-care-providers-should-publish-physician-ratings

223   **emails a twenty-question survey to every single patient** University of Utah Health Care. (2015). About the Press Ganey survey. http://healthcare.utah.edu/fad/pressganey.php

224   **We can begin to get data reporting right** Chatterjee, P., Tsai, T. C., & Jha, A. K. (2015). Delivering value by focusing on patient experience. *The American Journal of Managed Care, 21*(10), 735–737. www.ajmc.com/journals/issue/2015/2015-vol21-n910/delivering-value-by-focusing-on-patient-experience

226   **When the best practice for certain knee injuries** Skerrett, P. J. (2013). Physical therapy works as well as surgery for some with torn knee cartilage. Harvard Health Blog. *Harvard Health Publications, Harvard Medical School.* www.health.harvard.edu/blog/physical-therapy-works-as-well-as-surgery-for-some-with-torn-knee-cartilage-201303206002

228   **a doctors' strike tried to stop the Tommy Douglas government** Macdonald-Laurier Institute. (2014). Straight Talk: With Jeffrey Simpson. http://www.macdonaldlaurier.ca/files/pdf/SimpsonStraightTalk01-14-Draft4.pdf

229   **There is no requirement to participate in initiatives** Simpson, J. (2012). *Chronic Condition: Why Canada's Health Care System Needs to Be Dragged into the 21st Century.* Chapter 2: Health Care's Early History. Toronto: Penguin Group. http://onlinelibrary.wiley.com/doi/10.1111/capa.12046/abstract

230   **increasing its focus on the profession's social accountability** Health Canada. (2001). Social accountability: A vision for Canadian medical schools. www.afmc.ca/pdf/pdf_sa_vision_canadian_medical_schools_en.pdf

230   **training in areas like quality improvement** Baker, R. (2016). Quality improvement and patient safety. *Institute of Health Policy, Management and Evaluation, University of Toronto.* http://ihpme.utoronto.ca/academics/rd/qips-msc

230   **"the system" is something from which patients must be protected** Martin, D., & Whitehead, C. (2013). Physician, healthy system: The challenge of training doctor-citizens. *Medical Teacher, 35*(5), 416-417.

231   **"an embrace of citizenship . . ."** Berwick, D. M. (2009). The epitaph of profession. *British Journal of General Practice, 59*(559), 128–131. www.ncbi.nlm.nih.gov/pmc/articles/PMC2629825

231   **"Now you don your white coats . . ."** Berwick, D. M. (2012). To Isaiah. *Journal of the American Medical Association, 307*(24), 2597–2599. http://fhs.mcmaster.ca/surgery/isd/documents/GHJHToIsaiah.pdf

INDEX